AF300795

Psychopharmacology Series 11

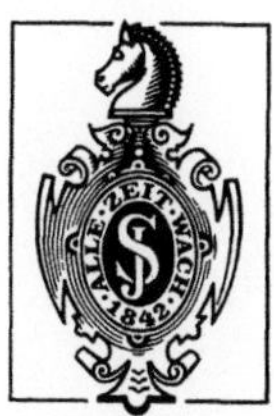

Anxiolytic β-Carbolines

From Molecular Biology to the Clinic

Editor

David N. Stephens

With 62 Figures, Some in Colour

Springer-Verlag

Berlin Heidelberg New York
London Paris Tokyo
Hong Kong Barcelona
Budapest

Dr. DAVID N. STEPHENS
Neuropsychopharmacology
Schering AG
Müllerstrasse 170-178
13353 Berlin
Germany

Cover illustration:
Model of the $GABA_A$ receptor complex

Vols. 1 and 2 of this series appeared under the title ,,Psychopharmacology Supplementum"

ISBN-13:978-3-642-78453-8   e-ISBN-13:978-3-642-78451-4
DOI: 10.1007/978-3-642-78451-4

Library of Congress Cataloging-in-Publication Data Anxiolytic [Beta]-carbolines : from molecular biology to the clinic / editor, David N. Stephens. p. cm. – (Psychopharmacology
series : v. 11) includes bibliographical references and index. ISBN-13:978-3-642-78453-8
1. Abecarnil – Testing. 2. Carbolines – Therapeutic use
– Testing. 3. GABA – Agonists – Therapeutic use – Testing. 4. Tranquilizing drugs –
Mechanisms of action. I. Stephens. David N., 1946 . II. Series. RM666.A12A56.1993
615'.7882 – dc20   93-33447

Typesetting: Best-set Typesetter Ltd., Hong Kong

25/3130/SPS-5 4 3 2 1 0 – Printed on acid-free paper

Preface

This monograph is the product of a symposium held in conjunction with the XVIIIth meeting of the Collegium Internationale Neuropsychologicum (CINP), held in Nice, France, in July 1992. In this symposium a large part of the available knowledge on abecarnil, a novel drug for treating anxiety disorders, was presented for the first time. In this volume the presentations at this symposium are supplemented by some additional chapters to provide a comprehensive overview of the pharmacology of the β-carboline abecarnil, from molecular biology to early clinical experiences, and a general introduction to the pharmacology of γ-aminobutyric acid type A ($GABA_A$) receptors and their interaction with different β-carbolines.

Abecarnil is a representative of the chemical class of β-carboline-3-carboxylic acid ester derivatives (shortened here for convenience to β-carbolines). The first compound of this class, β-carboline-3-carboxylic acid ethyl ester, was identified in human urine in a search for potential endogenous ligands for the then recently discovered brain benzodiazepine receptor. It quickly became clear that this substance was an artifact of the extraction procedure, but of significant importance was the observation that the pharmacological properties of the new compound differed from those of the benzodiazepines. Whereas the benzodiazepines possess anxiolytic, anticonvulsant, and muscle-relaxant properties, the new substance and its close derivatives gave rise to anxiety, induced convulsions, and enhanced muscle tone. Since it was already known that benzodiazepines achieve all their clinically useful effects by potentiating the action of the brain's major inhibitory transmitter, GABA, the new results pointed to the possibility of modulating GABAergic function in both positive and negative directions, and it was not long before other substances were discovered with intermediate abilities to modulate GABAergic transmission. These compounds, so-called partial agonists and partial inverse agonists at the benzodiazepine receptor, were recognized as potential novel drugs, and several pharmaceutical companies became involved in the search for partial agonists with anxiolytic potency but without the side effects of the classical benzodiazepines. Among these the Danish company A/S Ferrosan (now part of Novo-Nordisk) and the German company Schering AG concentrated their search among derivatives of β-carbolines. The discovery of β-carboline ligands for benzodiazepine receptors is described in the opening chapter by Claus Braestrup and Mogens Nielsen.

Although the β-carbolines were the first negative modulators of $GABA_A$-receptor function to be identified (unfortunately, for some less well informed pharmacologists, the term β-carboline is still practically synonymous with inverse agonist), it rapidly became clear that different compounds within the series covered the whole continuum of possible modulatory effects on $GABA_A$-receptor function. Indeed, the β-carboline series is probably the only chemical series which incorporates such a wide and continuous range of efficacies in modulating GABA function. The structure–activity relationships determining which compounds are inverse agonists and which are agonists are described in the chapter by Ralph Schmiechen and his colleagues.

The analysis of $GABA_A$-receptor function and the role of modulators of the $GABA_A$ receptor has been at the forefront of neuropharmacology for the last decade or more. Of particular importance was the emergence of the idea that a neurotransmitter receptor might be sensitive, not only to its own transmitter, but also to other agents capable of modifying its response to the transmitter. This principle, first elucidated for the $GABA_A$ receptor, has now been extended to another receptor-gated ion-channel complex, the N-methyl-D-aspartate (NMDA) receptor, and may represent a general principle of function of certain ligand-gated ion channel complexes. One of the most exciting aspects of this research has been the cloning of the $GABA_A$ receptor, the working out of its structure, and the discovery of a whole series of variations in its make up giving rise to several subtypes of receptor with different distributions in the brain, and showing quantitative and sometimes qualitative differences in their interactions with agents acting at benzodiazepine receptors. This pioneering work, carried out largely in the laboratories of Peter Seeburg and Eric Barnard, is described in the chapter by Seeburg's collaborator, Hartmut Lüddens. A complementary chapter by Jon Turner and coauthors describes the brain distribution of certain receptor components giving rise to receptor subtypes. The implications of this work for understanding the pharmacology of compounds like abecarnil are discussed by Iris Pribilla and her colleagues. Hitherto, although it has been found that certain compounds binding to benzodiazepine receptors show different affinities for different receptor subtypes, Pribilla demonstrates that abecarnil not only shows preferentially high affinity for certain receptor subtypes, but that the compound acts as a full agonist at certain subtypes and as a partial agonist at others. This is an exciting discovery which suggests the possibility of achieving very subtle manipulations of the clinical pharmacology of compounds acting at benzodiazepine receptor subtypes.

The theme introduced by Pribilla et al. in the context of recombinant receptors expressed in artificial conditions is taken up by the next two chapters. Giovanni Biggio's group demonstrate that despite abecarnil's selective in vivo action as an anxiolytic, the compound behaves as a full agonist at benzodiazepine receptors in biochemical pharmacological experiments in rat cortex; on the other hand, part of its in vivo action is typical of partial agonist activity. This is illustrated further in the chapter by Dai Stephens and colleagues, in which it is demonstrated that at those receptors at which abecarnil achieves its anxiolytic effects, abecarnil acts as a highly potent agonist. On the other hand, in tests of muscle relaxation, sedation, and ataxia, abecarnil behaves in a classical partial agonist fashion. These observations from animal pharmacology seem to reflect the compound's pharmacology at different recombinant receptor combinations, though it is clearly premature to attempt to ascribe a particular pharmacological function to abecarnil's action at particular subtypes of receptor.

These two chapters also serve to introduce the question of the development of dependence following chronic treatment with benzodiazepines. This is an issue which has found increasing public awareness over the last few years, and a major hope for novel and selective drugs acting at benzodiazepine receptors is that they might show less potential for inducing dependcence. Both Serra et al. and Stephens et al. present data suggesting advantages of abecarnil over standard benzodiazepines in this important aspect. This theme is taken up and expanded in the next three chapters by Wolfgang Löscher, Christine Sannerud and colleagues, and Michael Emmett-Oglesby's group. Löscher illustrates from his experiments with dogs that chronic treatment with abecarnil, in contrast to diazepam, does not lead to either the development of tolerance or to signs of dependence when the drug is withdrawn. This is largely confirmed by the work of Sannerud et al. using chronic treatment of baboons with high doses of abecarnil, and these authors also demonstrate that baboons do not self-administer abecarnil, in contrast to benzodiazepines such as triazolam. Whereas Löscher and Sannerud address the emergence of physical signs of dependence following withdrawal of drugs after chronic treatment, the chapter by Emmett-Oglesby investigates the subjective aspects of benzodiazepine withdrawal, using methods based on drug discrimination. Precipitation of withdrawal from abecarnil did not give rise to an internal stimulus resembling either withdrawal from chlordiazepoxide or the internal stimulus associated with administration of the anxiogenic drug pentylenetetrazole. Most provocatively, when rats were made dependent on a benzodiazepine and then switched to abecarnil for some days, no evidence of withdrawal reactions was seen, either during the switch to abecarnil or subsequently when abecarnil itself was withdrawn. If these sorts of observations can be extended to people, they would suggest not only a marked reduction in the dependence potential of abecarnil, but also that the drug might be used to wean dependent patients away from benzodiazepines.

The last chapter by Theodora Duka and coworkers brings the abecarnil story into the clinic. As well as documenting the first experiences of treating humans with abecarnil, this chapter describes the pharmacokinetics of the drug in healthy volunteers and the first evidence suggesting advantages of abecarnil over current benzodiazepines in terms of its effects on cognitive function. Lastly, this chapter addresses the first trial using abecarnil in the treatment of patients suffering from generalized anxiety disorder, in which the anxiolytic properties of the compound predicted from animal experimentation could be verified in the clinic.

I am grateful to the Chairman of the Organising Committee of the Collegium Internationale Neuropsychologicum, Professor G. Darcourt for his help in organising our symposium. Thanks also due to Drs. Steve Taylor and Matthias Suermondt, who through their organizational skills ensured a (more or less) stress-free symposium. Special thanks go to Manuela Weidmann for her efficient and friendly support, both during the organization of the meeting and in the preparation of this volume.

Berlin, October 1993   DAVID N. STEPHENS

Contents

List of Contributors

You will find the addresses at the beginning of the respective contribution

Discovery of β-Carboline Ligands for Benzodiazepine Receptors

C. Braestrup[1] and M. Nielsen[2]

The benzodiazepine class of drugs was discovered in the late 1950s by Sternbach and Randall at the Roche Laboratories in Basle, Switzerland. Until the mid-1980s all members of this pharmacological class were of a very similar nature chemically all being [1,4] benzodiazepine molecules (except clordiazepoxide, Fig. 1). Surprisingly, all new compounds discovered for almost three decades with the characteristic diazepam-like anxiolytic, hypnotic, and anticonvulsant profile were chemically classified as benzodiazepines. They were all remarkably similar in their clinical and pharmacological actions; they differed mainly with respect to potency, duration of action, existence of active metabolites, etc. The discovery of new chemical classes of compounds acting on benzodiazepine receptors, but not being [1,4] benzodiazepines, has broadened the pharmacodynamic profile of this class of drugs and has opened a new avenue for designing drugs with advantageous properties.

1 Mechanism of Action of Benzodiazepines

The first clues as to the way benzodiazepines work were obtained in 1975 when it was reported that they enhance the effect of the inhibitory neurotransmitter γ-aminobutyric acid (GABA; Haefely et al. 1975; Costa et al. 1975). GABA is the major inhibitory neurotransmitter in the mammalian central nervous system, and almost all effects of benzodiazepines can be explained by enhanced GABAergic function.

A more direct understanding of the mechanism of action of the benzodiazepine type of drugs was reached in 1977 when it was demonstrated that specific receptors exist for benzodiazepines on neurons in the central nervous system of all higher vertebrates (Squires and Braestrup 1977; Moehler and Okada 1977). These receptors were membrane proteins and were specifically localized in brain tissue where they were present on a great

[1] Pharmaceuticals Research, Novo Nordisk A/S, Novo Nordisk Park, DK-2760 Maaloev, Denmark
[2] Sct. Hans Mental Hospital, DK-4000 Roskilde, Denmark

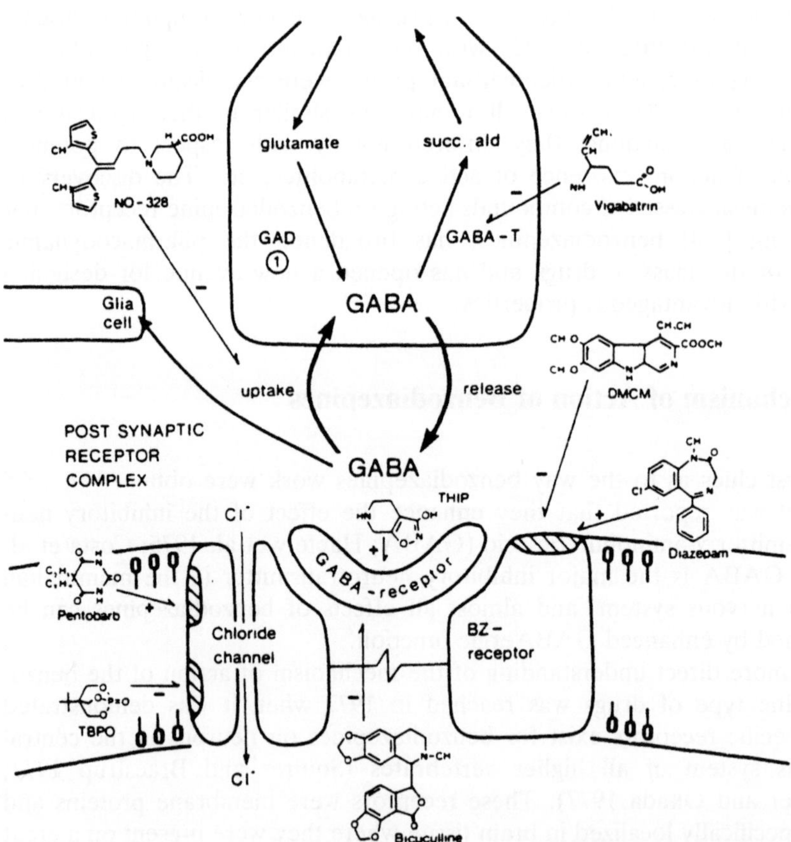

Fig. 1. Chemical structure of diazepam and β-carboline carboxylic acid ethyl ester (*β-CCE*). Both compounds show high affinity for benzodiazepine receptors (*K_i* values shown)

Fig. 2. A highly schematic diagram of the GABAergic synapse, showing the presynaptic terminal which releases GABA, and the postsynaptic membrane where GABA receptors and benzodiazepine receptors open chloride channels in concert. A number of targets are shown where drugs can affect the GABAergic neurotransmission

number of different kinds of neurons. In accordance with the clinical observation that benzodiazepines have very few peripheral side effects, peripheral tissues lacked benzodiazepine receptors. Benzodiazepine receptors
recognized all the clinically and pharmacologically active benzodiazepines,
and yet at the same time they showed remarkable selectivity, no other
known class of chemical compounds at that time showed any functionally
relevant affinity for these receptors.

In 1978 (Tallman et al. 1978) it became clear that the benzodiazepine
receptors and GABA receptors are intimately coupled at the molecular level
in a supramolecular GABA-receptor/benzodiazepine-receptor complex.
This complex provides the means for an allosteric interaction between
benzodiazepine receptors and GABA receptors, an interaction in which
benzodiazepines, when they occupy their receptors, enhance the function of
GABA receptors. GABA receptors in turn open channels for chloride flux
through the plasma membrane (Fig. 2).

The molecular nature of benzodiazepine and GABA receptors is now
known following the successful cloning and expression of the receptor
molecules (see Seeburg 1990). There is a whole family (more than 13
members) of very closely related receptor subtypes; the exact interplay of
which is not yet fully understood (see Luddens, this volume).

2 Elusive Endogenous Ligands for Benzodiazepine Receptors

Certainly one of the most intriguing questions relating to the benzodiazepine
receptor concerns the nature of its putative endogenous ligand. Benzodiazepine receptors must remain classified as drug receptors until the discovery of an endogenous agent (neurotransmitter or neuromodulator) which
exerts its effect via benzodiazepine receptors. The discovery of endogenous
ligands for opiate receptors was aided by the fact that appropriate bioassays,
such as the guinea pig ileum and in vitro receptor assays, were available for
testing for opiate activity in numerous samples during fractionation procedures. The discovery of benzodiazepine receptors initiated a similar search
for endogenous benzodiazepine-like endogenous factors; the ability of tissue
extracts to compete with radiolabelled benzodiazepines for their receptors
was used to detect the presence of putative ligands.

Many research groups embarked on purification from various biological
sources of agents with activity on benzodiazepine-receptor binding. Hypo-
xanthine and inosine were extracted from brain tissues and shown to have a
weak affinity for benzodiazepine receptors, also nicotinamide was isolated
by virtue of its affinity for benzodiazepine receptors, yet all of these compounds are generally believed not to be of physiological significance in
relation to benzodiazepine receptors. Another group of candidates, peptides
(DBI, ODN, and EP, see Gray et al. 1986), has attracted extensive interest.

Comprehensive literature exists describing these peptides in detail; they have been cloned and are found in specific neurons in the brain. DBI and ODN produce proconflict (anxiogenic?) responses after intraventricular injections into rats, furthermore, DBI is released by the depolarization of primary cultures of cortical neurons by potassium. While these properties certainly suggest a functional relation to the benzodiazepine receptor, several unresolved issues remain, and it is still unclear whether these peptide compounds are of actual physiological significance in the brain of living humans.

In 1979 it was reported that human urine contained a factor which possessed a remarkably high affinity for brain benzodiazepine receptors (Nielsen et al. 1979). Originally it was hypothesized that this factor represented urinary excretion of an endogenous ligand for benzodiazepine receptors or an active metabolite of such a ligand. The compound, called the gamma-fraction, was later identified as being β-carboline-3-carboxylic acid ethyl ester (β-CCE, see Fig. 1). The chemical nature of the isolated compound immediately revealed that this compound was not an endogenous ligand for benzodiazepine receptors because the ethyl ester grouping was evidently added artificially during the purification process. Furthermore, a search for enzymatic pathways which would lead from, for instance tryptophan, to the β-carboline, failed, which led to doubts that the β-carboline moiety actually has an important physiological function, since enzymatic pathways would be expected to regulate the synthesis and breakdown of important factors (Fig. 3).

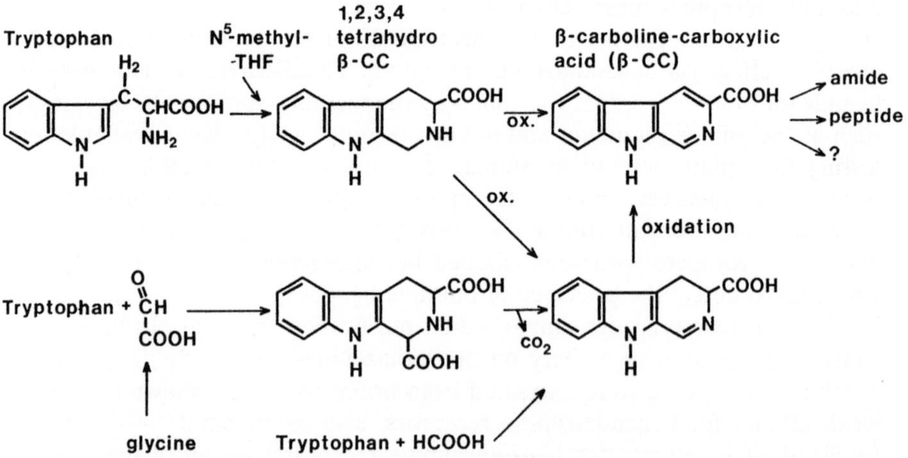

Fig. 3. Hypothetical pathways leading to β-carboline-3-carboxylic acid (*β-CC*). β-CC has a low affinity for benzodiazepine receptors ($K_i \simeq 15\,000\,\mathrm{nM}$)

Later, however, it has been hypothesized that the butyl ester of β-carboline-3-carboxylic acid (De Robertis et al. 1988) is an endogenous ligand for benzodiazepine receptors, but these studies have not been further corroborated.

While the β-carboline moiety thus may not be related to the still elusive endogenous ligand for benzodiazepine receptors, the β-carboline group of compounds has led to a new understanding of how benzodiazepine receptors function.

3 β-Carbolines as Ligands for Benzodiazepine Receptors with a Continuum of Efficacies

Surprisingly, it was discovered that β-carboline carboxylic acid ethyl ester did not produce the classical well-known hypnotic, sedative, and anticonvulsant effects of benzodiazepines in animals, yet the compound occupied benzodiazepine receptors in the living mouse brain. Even more surprisingly, it was discovered that a derivative of β-carboline carboxylic acid ethyl ester, DMCM (Fig. 2), produced frank convulsions in mice and rats (Braestrup et al. 1982). β-Carboline carboxylic acid ethyl ester, however, was able to antagonize both the benzodiazepine anticonvulsant effect and the convulsant effect of DMCM. These studies showed that the benzodiazepine receptor was capable of reacting in opposite directions depending on the nature of the ligand that bound the receptor. Anticonvulsant ligands like diazepam enhance the GABAergic function and produce anticonvulsant and other activity, while convulsant ligands such as DMCM reduce GABAergic function and produce their convulsant effects. In addition to being instrumental in the discovery that receptors can respond in opposite directions depending on the ligand that binds to it, the β-carboline was also capable of differentiating between various types of brain benzodiazepine receptors; β-carbolines seem to have a higher affinity for type I brain benzodiazepine receptors than type II brain benzodiazepine receptors (Nielsen and Braestrup 1980).

The fact that benzodiazepine receptors can respond in various directions depending on the nature of the ligand acting on the receptor led to the hypothesis that it would be possible to design compounds which had a selective affinity for the various subtypes of benzodiazepine receptors and at the same time showed just the right efficacy on these receptors thereby producing some of the beneficial effects of benzodiazepines, for example, the anxiolytic effects, while loosing other effects such as sedative effects and the development of tolerance. Abecarnil (see Stephens et al., this volume) is an example of a chemical optimization of the β-carboline nucleus to produce a compound with a finely selected profile of action.

References

Braestrup C, Nielsen M, Olsen CE (1980) Urinary and brain β-carboline-3-carboxylates as potent inhibitors of brain benzodiazepine receptors. Proc Natl Acad Sci USA 77:2288–2292

Braestrup C, Schmiechen R, Neef G, Nielsen M, Petersen EN (1982) Interaction of convulsive ligands with benzodiazepine receptors. Science 216:1241–1243

Costa E, Guidotti A, Mao CC, Suria A (1975) New concepts on the mechanism of action of benzodiazepines. Life Sci 17:167–186

De Robertis E, Pena C, Palandini AC, Medina JH (1988) New developments on the search for the endogenous ligands of central benzodiazepine receptors. Neurochem Int 13(1):1–12

Gray PW, Glaister D, Seeburg PH, Guidotti A, Costa E (1986) Cloning and expression of cDNA for human diazepam-binding inhibitor, a natural ligand of an allosteric regulatory site of the γ-aminobutyric acid type A receptor. Proc Natl Acad Sci USA 83:7547–7551

Haefely W, Kulcsar A, Moehler H, Pieri L, Polc P, Schaffner R (1975) Possible involvement of GABA in the central actions of benzodiazepines. In: Costa E, Greengard P (eds) Mechanism of action of benzodiazepines. Raven, New York, pp 131–151

Moehler H, Okada T (1977) Benzodiazepine receptors: demonstration in the central nervous system. Science 198:849–851

Nielsen M, Braestrup C (1980) Ethyl β-carboline-3-carboxylate shows differential benzodiazepine-receptor interaction. Nature 286:606–607

Nielsen M, Gredal O, Braestrup C (1979) Some properties of ^{3}H-diazepam displacing activity from human urine. Life Sci 25:679–686

Squires RF, Braestrup C (1977) Benzodiazepine receptors in rat brain. Nature 266: 732–734

Seeburg PH, Wisden W, Verdoorn TA, Pritchett DB, Werner P, Herb A, Lueddens H, Sprengel R, Sakmann B (1990) The GABA. A receptor family molecular and functional diversity. In: The brain. Cold Spring Harbor Laboratory Press, New York, pp 29–40 (Cold Spring Harbor Symposia on Quantitative Biology, vol 55)

Tallman JF, Thomas JW, Gallager DW (1978) GABAergic modulation of benzodiazepine binding-site sensitivity. Nature 274:383–385

β-Carboline-3-Carboxylic Acid Ethyl Ester: a Lead for New Psychotropic Drugs

R. Schmiechen[1], D. Seidelmann, and A. Huth

1 Introduction

Beta-carboline-3-carboxylic-acid ethyl ester (β-CCE) was isolated by Claus Braestrup while he was searching for the endogenous ligand of the benzodiazepine receptor (BZ receptor). Although this compound was not the endogenous ligand but an artifact of the isolation procedure, it was considered a promising lead for the development of psychotropic drugs acting via the BZ receptor because of the following features:

- High affinity (better than diazepam)
- Partial selectivity for specific brain areas (in contrast to BZs)
- Pharmacological effects mediated by the BZ receptor but differing from BZs (antagonistic or even partial inverse agonistic)
- A rather simple chemical structure permitting a vast number of modifications

It was predicted that optimisation of this lead would result in drug compounds exhibiting a dissociation of the complex pharmacological profile seen in the classical BZs of the 1960s and 1970s, combined with a better metabolic stability than β-CCE itself.

2 Optimising Affinity for Benzodiazepine Receptors

The basis for the planned modifications of the lead structure aiming at profile dissociation and metabolic stability was to be discovery of the structural requirements for high receptor affinity. Thus the primary target of the optimisation project – jointly undertaken in the Research Laboratories of Schering and Ferrosan – were drastic variations of the β-carboline skeleton to elucidate the essential parts of the molecule for high receptor-binding activity. As a first step, hydrogenation as well as ring opening (Fig. 1) was studied.

---

[1] Research Laboratories of Schering AG, 13342 Berlin, Germany

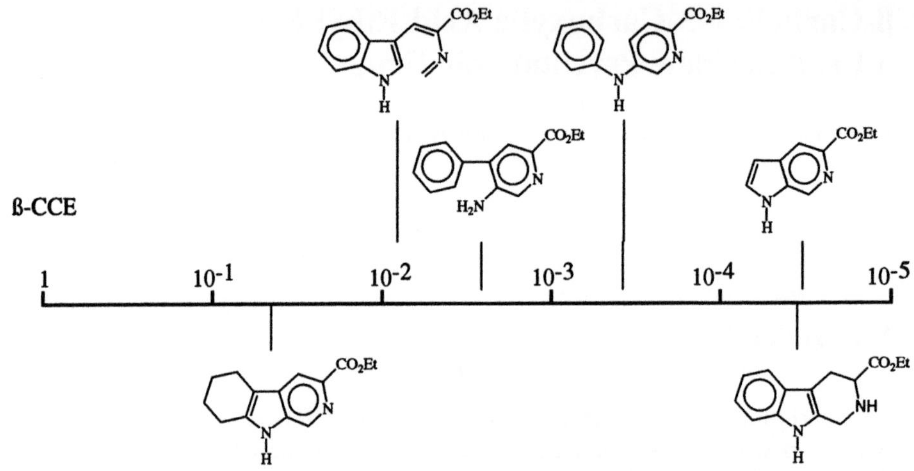

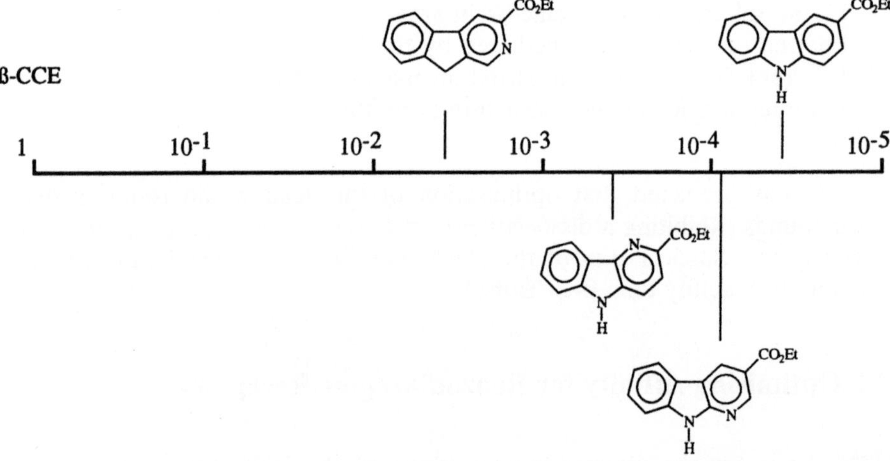

Fig. 1. The effects of hydrogenisation and ring opening of the β-CCE molecule on the relative affinity for ^{3}H-flunitrazepam-labelled receptors. β-CCE (IC_{50} = 2.5 nM) has been allocated a value of 1, and the affinity of the structural variations expressed proportionately

Fig. 2. The effect of varying the position of the C ring nitrogen, or of replacing it with a carbon atom on the relative affinity for ^{3}H-flunitrazepam-labelled receptors: β-CCE (IC_{50} = 2.5 nM) has been allocated a value of 1, and the affinity of the structural variations expressed proportionately

Both variations led to a 100–10000-fold decrease in receptor affinity, clearly pointing to the essential nature of the complete aromatic carboline system. An exception is the partial hydrogenation of the carbon-ring, which reduces the binding capacity by only a factor of 20.

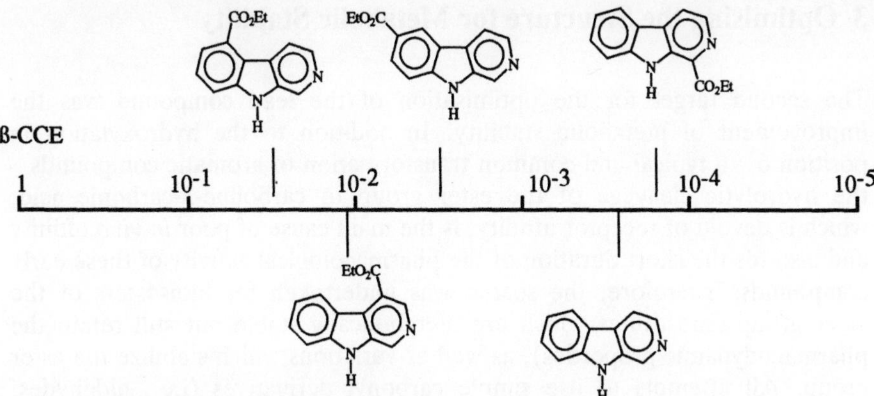

Fig. 3. Effect of varying the position of the ester moiety on the relative affinity for ^{3}H-flunitrazepam-labelled receptors. β-CCE (IC_{50} = 2.5 nM) has been allocated a value of 1, and the affinity of the structural variations expressed proportionately

Shifting the nitrogen from position 2 (β) to 1 (α) or 4 (δ) or replacement of one or the other nitrogen by carbon also leads to an dramatic loss of affinity (Fig. 2).

Comparison of isomeric β-carboline-ethyl carboxylates clearly demonstrates the 3 position as the optimal site for the ester moiety (Fig. 3).

The remarkably low affinity of the 1-carbonic acid ester – even lower than that of the unsubstituted β-carboline – furnished the first hint on topological requirements for optimal receptor fit, and led to the hypothesis that substitution in the lower part of the molecule interferes severely with receptor fit. This assumption could be substantiated by replacing, step by step, every hydrogen atom by a fluorine atom or a methyl group. A comparison of these derivatives with the unsubstituted lead compound revealed only a marginal influence on receptor affinity of variations in position 4,5 or 6, a medium decrease in position 7, but a dramatic loss (100- to 5000-fold) in positions 1,8 or 9.

Without exception this characteristic influence of the substitution pattern could be demonstrated for a variety of other substituents differing in size as well as physicochemical properties (Fig. 4).

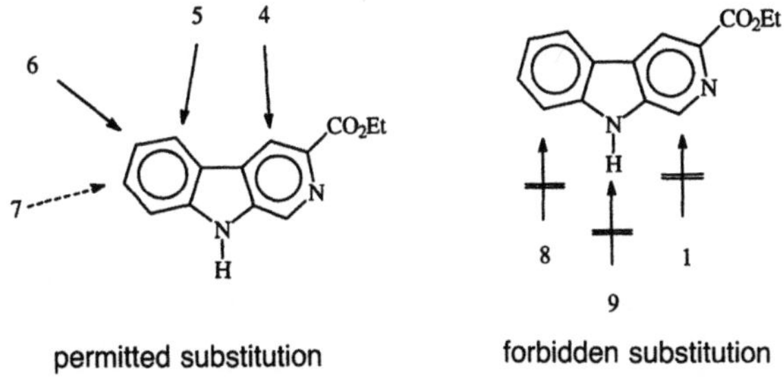

Fig. 4. Summary of substitution patterns maintaining or drastically reducing affinity for benzodiazepine receptors

3 Optimising the Structure for Metabolic Stability

The second target for the optimisation of the lead compound was the improvement of metabolic stability. In addition to the hydroxylation in position 6 – a typical and common transformation of aromatic compounds – the hydrolytic cleavage of the ester group to carboline-3-carbonic acid, which is devoid of receptor affinity, is the main cause of poor *in vivo* affinity and also for the short duration of the pharmacological activity of these early compounds. Therefore, the search was undertaken for bioisosters of the ester group (substitutes which are metabolically stable but still retain the pharmacodynamic properties), as well as variations which stabilize the ester group. All attempts to use simple carbonyl derivatives (i.e., aldehydes, ketones, amides, and nitriles) as bioisosters were disappointing in respect to affinity and/or stability but some heterocycles especially oxadiazoles, proved to be perfect bioisosters (Hansen et al. 1986).

Although first discovered with β-carbolines, the use of oxadiazoles as bioisosteric equivalents to the ester group is not limited to this class as could be demonstrated by application of this principle to other classes of drugs, e.g. benzodiazepines and muscarinergic agents (Jensen et al. 1988; Wätjen et al. 1989; Street et al. 1990). The use of these bioisosters has subsequently found wide acceptance in other areas of drug discovery (Schönafinger and Bohn 1987; Swain et al. 1991). An alternative way improving the metabolic stability of the lead compound was to protect the ester moiety against attack of esterases by steric hindrance (i.e. substitution by more or less bulky groups close to the reactive centre of the carbonic acid ester, the carbonyl group) (Fig. 5).

Since the ester group is essential for high receptor affinity, manipulation close to this centre may imply an deleterious effect on the binding properties. Examining different variations of R_4 and R_1 revealed the critical

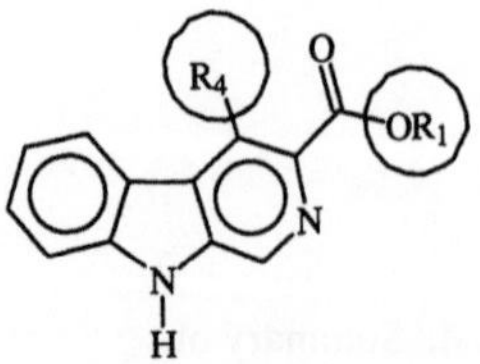

Fig. 5. Metabolic stability is improved through protection of the ester moiety by steric hindrance. (R_4, lower alkyl, substituted alkyl (i.e. CH_2OCH_3); R_1, i-propyl, t-butyl, i-butyl)

spatial situation with respect to receptor affinity especially in position 4, which does not allow the use of highly branched alkyl groups. Thus protection of the ester group without effect on receptor affinity is optimally achieved by moderate shielding in both positions.

4 General Rules for Structural Optimisation of β-Carbolines

A consideration of all the results of systematic variations of β-CCE undertaken to find relations between chemical structure and receptor affinity as well as to stability led to a refined lead structure suitable for optimising the pharmacological profile, and particularly the dissociation of the typical BZ activity profile into its component parts (Fig. 6). This structure can be described as follows:

– A full aromatic plane β-Carboline system
– No substitution in positions 1,8 and 9
– A metabolically stable ester group or a bioisoster in position 3
– Open to a wide range of substitution in positions 5 and 6
– Limited freedom of substitution in position 4 and 7

Compound finding based on the refined lead structure revealed a large number of pharmacologically interesting compounds covering the entire activity spectrum ranging from agonists with the complete profile of BZ-agonist such as lorazepam, through partial agonists and mixed agonist/

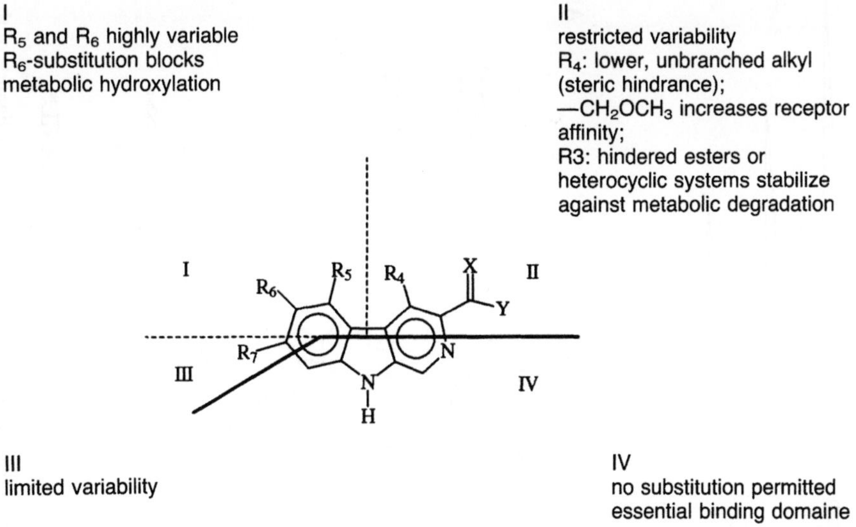

Fig. 6. Summary of allowed and prohibited substitutions of the β-carboline structure leading to changes in affinity and/or metabolic stability

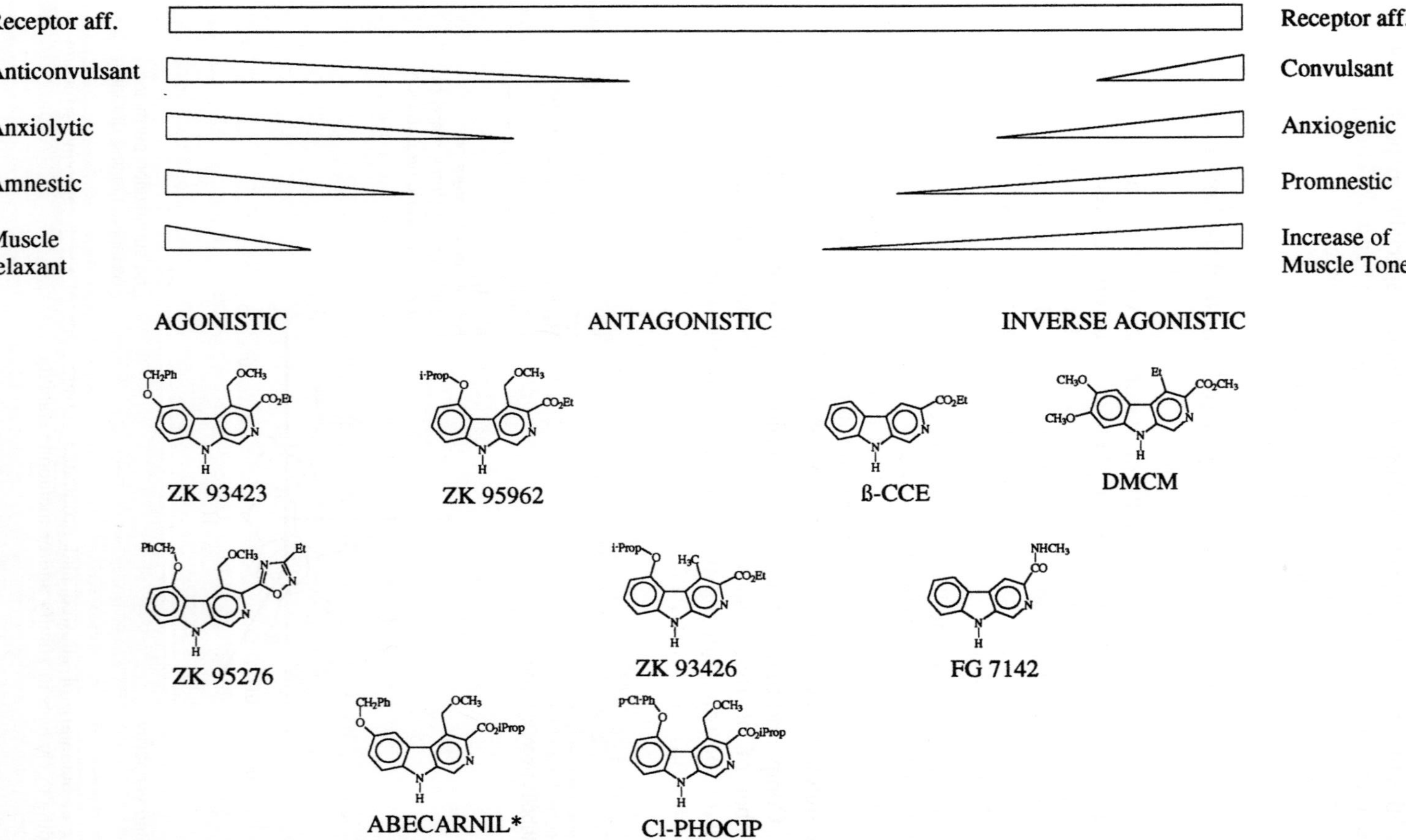

Fig. 7. The position of some typical BZ receptor ligands of the β-carboline family. *Asterisk* indicates that abecarnil does not fit completely to this scheme (*Et*, C_2H_5; *i-Prop*, $CH(CH_3)_2$; *Ph*, C_6H_5; *p-Cl-Ph*, $4\text{-}Cl\text{-}C_6H_4$)

antagonists, to pure BZ antagonists without any direct pharmacological activity. Besides the partial agonists, which already show the aspired improved profile, compounds have also been identified and characterised which are described best as selective agonists. One representative of this type is the nonsedating and nonmuscle relaxant, abecarnil (Duka et al. 1993).

Surprisingly, β-carboline derivatives have also been identified that exhibit negative efficacy combined with high receptor affinity – a unique phenomenon not previously known from the pharmacology of any other receptor system. These compounds showing the exact mirror image of the effects of BZ agonists have been called inverse agonists and turned out to be valuable tools for the characterisation of the BZ-binding site and the understanding of the function of GABA-mediated neurotransmission. The convulsant DMCM is a typical representative of this group. As well as offering valuable pharmacological tools, inverse agonists and partial or selective inverse agonists may open an avenue to new drugs which could be beneficial for the treatment of memory and other cognitive disorders (Sarter and Stephens 1988; Stephens et al. 1991). The position of some typical BZ receptor ligands of the β-carboline family within the extended spectrum of ligands ranging from agonists to inverse agonists is shown in Fig. 7.

The location of these derivatives in the diagram is based on their biochemical and pharmacological characterisation and has been fully confirmed (with the exception of β-CCE and DMCM) by human trials in volunteers and in part in patients (Dorow et al. 1983, 1987; Duka et al. 1990; Möller et al. 1990).

The basic relationships between chemical structure and pharmacological activity derived from the most intensively characterised compounds (Fig. 7) have been confirmed by the pharmacological profile of numerous other β-carboline derivatives. Generally an increase in efficacy, i.e. a shift to a more agonistic profile, is caused by the following variations:

– Increase of lipophilicity of substituents in position 5 or 6.

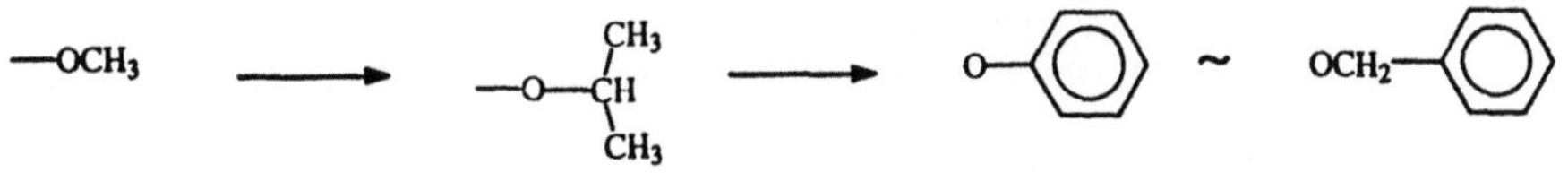

– Shift of a given substituent from position 5 to position 6.

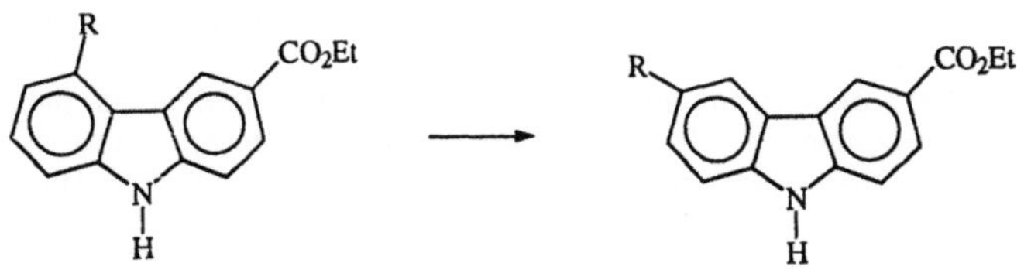

– Replacement of lower alkyl in position 4 by the $-CH_2OCH_3$-group which additionally improves the receptor affinity.

$$-CH_3 \; , \quad -C_2H_5 \quad \longrightarrow \quad -CH_2OCH_3$$

– Exchange of the 3-carbonic ester group by bio-isosteric equivalents, e.g., oxadiazoles.

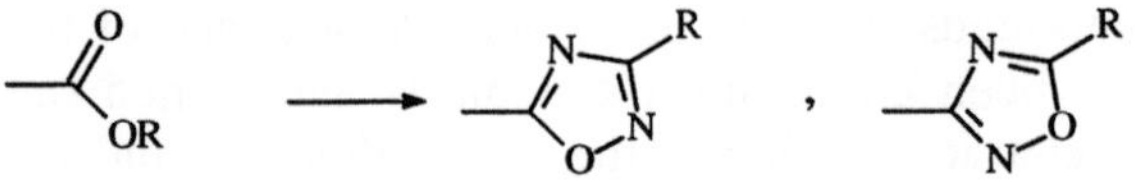

Interestingly, the typical agonist shift induced by substituting an oxadiazole moiety for an ester function is not limited to β-carbolines, but is also seen in the benzodiazepine series (Hansen et al. 1986).

Acknowledgement. The authors wish to acknowledge the collaboration and support of our colleagues in chemistry, biochemistry and pharmacology at A/S Ferrosan and Schering AG.

References

Dorow R, Duka T, Höller L, Sauerbrey N (1987) Clinical perspectives of β-carbolines from first studies in humans. Brain Res Bull 19(3):319–326

Dorow R, Horowski R, Paschelke G, Amin M, Braestrup C (1983) Severe anxiety induced by FG 7142, a β-carboline ligand for benzodiazepine receptors. Lancet II:98

Duka T, Stephens DN, Dorow R (1990) Cognitive enhancing properties of antagonist β-carbolines: New insights into clinical research on the treatment of dementias? In: Maurer K, Riederer P, Beckmann H (eds) Alzheimer's disease. Epidemiology, neuropathology, neurochemistry and clinics. Springer, Berlin, Heidelberg, New York, Tokyo, pp 555–564

Duka T, Schütt B, Krause W, Dorow R, Mc Donald S, Fichte K (1993) Human studies on Abecarnil a new β-carboline anxiolytic: safety, tolerability and preliminary pharmacological profile. Br J Clin Pharmacol 35:386–394

Hansen JB, Engelstoft M, Honore T, Wätjen F, Schmiechen R (1986) 3-(1,2,4-Oxadiazolyl-β-carboline) derivates as benzodiazepine receptor ligands. IXth International Symposium on Medical Chemistry, Berlin

Jensen LH, Wätjen F, Honoré T, Hansen JB, Engelstoft M, Schmiechen R (1988) Oxadiazolylimidazobenzodiazepines: new class of benzodiazepine receptor ligands. In: Briggs G, Casta E (eds) Chloride channels and their modulation by neurotransmitters and drugs. Raven, New York

Möller A, Jensen LM, Skrumsager B, Blatt-Lyon B, Pederson B, Dam M (1990) Inhibition of photosensitive seizures in man by the β-carboline, ZK 95962, a selective benzodiazepine receptor agonist. Epilepsy Res 5:155–159

Sarter M, Stephens DN (1988) Beta-carbolines as tools in memory research: animal data and speculations. In: Hindmarch I, Ott H (eds) Benzodiazepine receptor ligands: memory and information processing. Springer, Berlin Heidelberg New York (Psychopharmacology Series, vol 9) pp 230–245

Schönafinger K, Bohn M (1987) Synthese und Ca-antagonistische Wirkung eines chiralen Dihydropyridins. GDCH, Schweizer Chemische Gesellschaft: neuere Entwicklungen in der medizinischen Chemie: Agonisten und Antagonisten an Ionenkanälen, Freiburg, September 6–9

Stephens DN, Duka T, Andrews JS (1991) Benzodiazepines, β-carbolines and memory. In: Weinman J, Hunter J (eds) Memory: neurochemical and abnormal perspectives. Harwood, London

Street LJ, Baker R, Book T, Kneen CO, Macleod AM, Merchant KJ, Showell GA, Saunders J, Herbert R, Freedman SB, Harley EA (1990) Synthesis and biological activity of 1,2,4-oxadiazole derivates: highly potent and efficacious agonist for cortical muscarine receptors. J Med Chem 33:2690–2697

Swain CJ, Baker R, Kneen C, Moseley I, Saunders J, Seward EM, Stevenson G, Beer M, Stanton J, Watling H (1991) Novel 5-HT$_3$ antagonist: indole oxadiazoles. J Med Chem 34:140–151

Wätjen F, Baker R, Engelstoft M, Herbert R, Macleod AM, Knight A, Merchant KJ, Moseley J, Saunders J, Swain CJ, Wong E, Springe J (1989) Novel benzodiazepine receptor partial agonists: oxadiazolylimidazobenzodiazepines. J Med Chem 32: 2282–2291

Molecular Biology of Gamma-Aminobutyric Acid Type A/Benzodiazepine Receptors

H. LÜDDENS

1 Architecture of Ligand-Gated Ion Channels

Ligand-gated ion channels mediate large parts of the fast synaptic neuro-transmission in the central nervous system (Dingledine et al. 1988). In recent years, mainly as a result of modern molecular-biology techniques, the understanding of the pharmacology, biochemistry, and electrophysiology of these channels has advanced greatly. The family of ligand-gated ion channels now comprises the molecularly related nicotinic acetylcholine receptors (AChR), the γ-aminobutyric acid type A receptors (GABA$_A$R), the glycine receptors (GlyR), the serotonin receptor 5-hydroxytryptamin$_3$ (5-HT$_3$), and possibly some receptors of the glutamate receptor family (GluR; Betz 1990; Maricq et al. 1991; Monyer et al. 1992; Moriyoshi et al. 1991; Schofield et al. 1987).

The structural feature common to most ligand-gated ion channels/ receptors (AChR, GABA$_A$R, GlyR, and 5-HT$_3$) is the four membrane-spanning domains, present in each of the different subunits. The presumed five subunits (Unwin 1989) arrange around the central channel pore, the gating of which is controlled by the respective neurotransmitters. Polar but uncharged amino acid positions are conserved in the second transmembrane helices (TM2) of the proteins belonging to the superfamily (Betz 1990; Unwin 1989). These amino acids may form the inner lining of the pores, thus providing the hydrophilic environment essential for the selectivity and passage of ions (Unwin 1989). Little is known about the arrangement and function of the other three transmembrane domains.

All members of the superfamily (apart from the GluR) contain two cysteine residues that are separated by 13 amino acids in the N-terminal extracellular domain (Fig. 1). For the nAChR the two cysteine residues are thought to form the "cys-cys loop" (Kao and Karlin 1986; Mosckovitz and Gershoni 1988) essential for certain aspects of the tertiary structure, a feature that is likely to extend to other members of the superfamily. The generally agreed upon sequence of the cys-cys-loop is conserved for most

Laboratory for Molecular Neuroendocrinology, Center for Molecular Biology, Im Neuen-heimer Feld 282, 69120 Heidelberg, Germany

```
      rat α1    QAECPMHLEDFPMDAHSCPLK
      rat α2    RAECPMHLEDFPMDAHACPLK
      rat α3    HAECPMHLEDFPMDVHACPLK
      rat α4    SAECPMRLVDFPMDGHACPLK
      rat α5    SAECPMQLEDFPMDAHACPLK
      rat α6    NADCPMRLVNFPMDGHACPLK
   rat β1,2,3   TAACMMDLRR[YP]LDEQNCTLE
   chicken β4   TAACMMDLRR[YP]LDQQNCTLE
      rat δ     TVACDMDLAK[YP]MDEQECMLD
      rat γ1    NAECYLQLHNFPMDEHSCPLE
      rat γ2    DAECQLQLHNFPMDEHSCPLE
      rat γ3    NAECQLQLHNFPMDAHACPLT
     human ρ1   TAMCNMDFSRFPLDTQTCSLE
   rat GlyR α1  TLACPMDLKNFPMDVQTCIMQ
   rat GlyR β   TLSCPLDLTLFPMDTQRCKMQ
   rat 5-HT₃    VTACSLDIYNFPFDVQNCSLT
   rat nACh α1  KSYCEIIVTHFPFDEQNCSMK
   rat nACh α2  KSSCSIDVTFFPFDQQNCKMK
   rat nACh β2  KSACKIEVKHFPFDQQNCTMK

   CONSENSUS  ---C------FP-D---C---
```

Fig. 1. Sequence comparison of the N-terminal, extracellular cysteine-cysteine loops of GABA$_A$-receptor subunits, the α_1- and β-glycine (*GlyR*) subunits, the 5-hydroxytryptamin$_3$ (*5-HT$_3$*) receptor, and the nicotinic acetylcholine (*nACh*) receptor subunits α_1, α_2, and β_2. All sequences are shown in the one letter code. The consensus sequence of conserved amino acid positions is shown in the last line. The deviation of the four β and the δ subunits from the consensus sequence is *boxed*. The references for the sequences are given in the text

members of the family, excluding the β and the δ subunits. In these two classes a tyrosine replaces a phenylalanine (Fig. 1). This holds true regardless of whether the sequences are derived from chicken or mammalian sources.

The described common structural elements apply to at least the "inner circle" of the superfamily of the ligand-gated ion channels (AChR, GABA$_A$R, GlyR, and 5-HT$_3$), but it has not yet been resolved whether similar elements are found within the group of GluR. The four former receptors display the common characteristics though they respond to four different ligands and are either cation (AChR, 5-HT$_3$) or anion selective (GABA$_A$R, GlyR).

GABA and glycine are the main inhibitory neurotransmitters in the central nervous system (CNS). Whereas GlyR are concentrated in the brain stem and the spinal cord, the GABA$_A$R are the most abundant inhibitory-acting channels in the remaining parts of the CNS. The question arises as to how a single type of receptor can fulfill its regulatory tasks in the diverse settings of the higher brain regions.

2 Subunit Heterogeneity

Most families in the group of the ligand-gated ion channels are multimembered. Their diversity provides a means to build a large array of different receptors from a limited number of proteins. The $GABA_AR$ is no exception to this rule.

2.1 Diversity of Subunits

Originally the $GABA_AR$ were thought to consist of two different subunits, named α and β according to the pattern in SDS PAGE of receptors purified from bovine brain (Sigel et al. 1983). Early pharmacological and biochemical data provided clues to the existence of receptor subtypes, but the diversity of $GABA_AR$ subunits was not anticipated until the cloning of the 15 different proteins detected in the mammalian CNS and the retina (Cutting et al. 1991; Lüddens and Wisden 1991; Seeburg et al. 1990). Using the amino acid sequence as a guide line, the subunits were grouped into five classes with one to six variants (α_{1-6}, β_{1-3}, γ_{1-3}, δ, and ρ_1) according to the degree of amino acid identity. One further β subunit was identified in chick brain (β_4; Bateson et al. 1991). Whereas the first four classes ($\alpha-\delta$) constitute classical $GABA_ARs$, functional proof for membership is missing for the ρ_1 variant (Shimada et al. 1992). Though originally an arbitrary classification, the amino acid identity measure turned out to reflect functional similarities as well.

Two subunits further contribute to the subunit diversity in that they exist in splice variants (Bateson et al. 1991; Kufuji et al. 1991; Whiting et al. 1990). The best studied example is the $\gamma_{2'}$ form that contains an eight amino-acid-long insert between transmembrane regions 3 and 4 (TM3 and TM4) as compared to the γ_2 variant, adding a potential phosphorylation site to the γ_2 subunit. It has been proposed that this site is involved in the ethanol sensitivity of $GABA_AR$ expressed in *Xenopus* oocytes (Wafford et al. 1991). The chicken β_4 subunit exists in two forms (β_4 and $\beta_{4'}$) that differ by a 12 base pair long insert, again into the intracellular loop between TM3 and TM4 (Bateson et al. 1991).

Even without taking into account the diversity added by the splice variants and the ρ_1 subunit, 72 $GABA_AR$ combinations of the form $\alpha_{x2}\beta_{x2}\gamma_x$ or $\alpha_{x2}\beta_{x2}\delta$ may exist in the mammalian brain. If one considers the possibility of different variants of one class in a single receptor, e.g., $\alpha_x\alpha_y\beta_x\beta_y\gamma_x$, or other subunit stoichiometries, e.g., $\alpha_{x3}\beta_{x2}$, the theoretical number of different receptors increases many times. However, further assumptions restrict the theoretical number. One important restriction is based on the subunit codistribution in the brain.

2.2 Distribution of the Subunits in the Brain

Most of the information we have gained on the GABA$_A$R distribution in the brain is based on in situ hybridization data of subunit mRNA in the rat brain. The mRNA coding for α_{1-6}, β_{1-3}, γ_{1-3}, and δ all display unique distribution in the mammalian CNS, but some neuronal cell populations, such as the dentate granule cells, contain all mRNA species besides the α_6 mRNA (Laurie et al. 1992; Wisden et al. 1992). Other areas, such as the Purkinje cells of the cerebellum, express only a limited number of GABA$_A$R mRNAs (Laurie et al. 1992; Shivers et al. 1989).

The α_1 mRNA is the most prominent GABA$_A$R subunit in the rodent brain and is widely codistributed with the β_2 mRNA (Khrestchatisky et al. 1989; Laurie et al. 1992; Malherbe et al. 1990b; Sequier et al. 1988; Wisden et al. 1992). The γ_2 variant mRNA often colocalizes with these two mRNA species (Laurie et al. 1992; Malherbe et al. 1990b; Shivers et al. 1989; Wisden et al. 1992). This triple combination constitutes the vast majority of GABA$_A$R mRNA in a number of cell populations. On the other hand, $\alpha_1\beta_2\gamma_1$ as well as $\alpha_1\beta_2\gamma_2$ receptors may assemble from the mRNA combinations present in the globus pallidus (Laurie et al. 1992; Wisden et al. 1992; Ymer et al. 1990).

$\alpha_2\beta_3$ and $\alpha_5\beta_1$ combinations are the most abundant GABA$_A$R mRNA species in the hippocampus (Laurie et al. 1992; Wisden et al. 1992) and may form the majority of the GABA$_A$Rs in this brain area with or without an additional γ_x variant.

The δ subunit mRNA is colocalized in large parts of the thalamus with mRNA that codes for the α_1, α_4, and β_2 subunits, whereas the γ_x mRNAs are virtually absent (Laurie et al. 1992; Shivers et al. 1989; Wisden et al. 1992). In the cerebellar granule cells the δ mRNA is present together with α_1, α_6, and β_2 mRNA, but in these cells substantial amounts of γ_2 mRNA can be detected (Laurie et al. 1992; Lüddens et al. 1990; Shivers et al. 1989). Thus, $\alpha_1(\alpha_4, \alpha_6)\beta_2\delta$ receptors may be formed (Wisden et al. 1992), but other options, like $\alpha_4\delta$ in the thalamus or $\alpha_6\delta$ in the cerebellum, cannot be excluded, especially in view of the close sequence identity of the β and the δ subunits (compare Fig. 1).

Little information is available on the distribution of the proteins corresponding to the mRNAs. The intracellular location of a mRNA in a neuron may drastically differ from the area where the protein inserts into the plasma membrane. Therefore the pattern of the protein and the corresponding mRNA distribution may differ. For a number of subunits and for most parts of the brain, the two distribution patterns overlap (Benke et al.

1991; Laurie et al. 1992; Shivers et al. 1989; Wisden et al. 1992; Zimprich et al. 1991), leaving only a few exceptions like the intensities of the γ_2 signals in the hippocampus which is high for the mRNA signal but low for the immunoreactivity (Malherbe et al. 1990b; Shivers et al. 1989; Wisden et al. 1992).

3 Role of Subunits

3.1 Subunit Composition of GABA$_A$R

Coexpression of the α_1 and β_1 subunits in *Xenopus laevis* oocytes resulted in Cl^- channels opened by GABA (Schofield et al. 1987) as was expected from the original biochemical data showing the copurification of two protein bands on a benzodiazepine (BZ)-affinity column (Sigel et al. 1983). Furthermore, the α_2, α_3, and α_5 variants coexpressed in *X. laevis* oocytes with β_1, and α_1 together with β_1, β_2, or β_3 all assemble to GABA-gated ion channels (Levitan et al. 1988; Ymer et al. 1989 a,b). The exchange of one α variant for another in an $\alpha_x\beta_1$ combination shifted the dose-response curve for GABA, but it did not affect the overall pharmacological properties of the resulting channels (Levitan et al. 1988). These heteromeric recombinant GABA channels were positively modulated by pentobarbital and blocked by picrotoxin and bicuculline, classifying them as GABA$_A$R. However, early studies (Schofield et al. 1987), more recently confirmed (Malherbe et al. 1990a), showed that the GABA response of *X. laevis* oocytes expressing $\alpha_1\beta_1$ subunits was only inconsistently modified by BZs.

3.2 BZ Receptors

Only when the γ_2 subunit was coexpressed in the human embryonic kidney cell line 293 with an α and a β variant, were GABA$_A$ channels formed, which consistently responded to BZ ligands, i.e., the receptors resembled the GABA$_A$/BZ receptors described for the mammalian brain (Pritchett et al. 1989). The γ_2 subunit is the most abundant member of the γ class in rat brain, with the other two variants being rarely expressed (Herb et al. 1992; Knoflach et al. 1991; Shivers et al. 1989; Ymer et al. 1990). Moreover, no biochemical or pharmacological evidence indicates the existence of γ_3-containing receptors in vivo. The coexpression of the α_1, β_2, and γ_3 in 293 cells leads to GABA$_A$R recognizing BZ ligands with reduced affinities for agonistic-acting (Table 1) BZ ligands as compared to antagonists or inverse agonists (Herb et al. 1992; Knoflach et al. 1991). Replacing the γ_2 with a γ_1 subunit in an $\alpha_x\beta_x\gamma_x$ combination (Ymer et al. 1990) leaves BZ receptors with a pharmacology reminiscent of the peripheral type BZ acceptor site (Lueddens and Skolnick 1987).

Table 1. Effect of different classes of central BZ ligands on GABA-stimulated channel function of $\alpha_x\beta_x\gamma_2$ receptors

	Synonym	Cl$^-$ flux	Example
+ Modulator	Agonist	Increase	Diazepam, flunitrazepam
− Modulator	Inverse agonist	Decrease	β-CCM Ro 15-4513
Antagonist	Blocker	No effect	Flumazenil

+, positive; −, negative

3.2.1 GABA$_A$/BZ Type I and II Receptors

It has long been apparent that heterogeneity exists in BZ-binding sites associated with the GABA$_A$ complex. Three lines of evidence supported this notion. Photolabeling experiments with [^{3}H]flunitrazepam and [^{3}H]Ro 15-4513 revealed the presence of several proteins with unique sizes and tryptic patterns (Eichinger and Sieghart 1985; Hebebrand et al. 1986; Sieghart and Karobath 1980). Furthermore, autoradiographic studies on rat-brain sections indicate mismatches between the binding of GABA$_A$R ligands, different BZ ligands, and convulsants such as TBPS (Olsen and Tobin 1990). Most BZ bind to the GABA$_A$/BZ receptors with similar affinities throughout the brain, but the binding properties of several compounds, most notably Cl 218 872 (Nielsen and Braestrup 1980; Sieghart 1983; Squires et al. 1979) and 2-oxoquazepam (Corda et al. 1988), demonstrated the heterogeneity of GABA$_A$/BZ receptors. Type I receptors have greater affinity with the triazolopyridine Cl 218 872 than type II receptors and constitute the predominant GABA$_A$R class in the CNS. The lower affinity type II receptors are enriched in hippocampus, striatum, and spinal cord (Lo et al. 1983; Sieghart et al. 1985).

Coexpression of the α_1, β_1, and γ_2 subunits in 293 cells leads to the assembly of functional GABA$_A$R that display the characteristics of BZ type I receptors (Pritchett et al. 1989). Exchange of the β_1 by any other β variant does not alter the affinity of any BZ ligand to the receptor complex (Pritchett et al. 1989). However, the K_a of the channel for GABA and the current modulation by diazepam are changed when the β_2 subunit is replaced by β_1 in a *X. laevis* expression system (Sigel et al. 1990). On the other hand, replacing the α_1 subunit with any other α variant dramatically affects the affinity of the formed GABA$_A$/BZ-receptor complex to selected BZ ligands (Pritchett et al. 1989; Table 2).

Whereas the pharmacological and electrophysiological properties of the GABA$_A$/BZ I receptors can only be mimicked by recombinant receptors of the $\alpha_1\beta_x\gamma_2$ type, BZ II receptors assemble in 293 cells from the α_2, α_3, or α_5 variants together with the $\beta_x\gamma_2$ combination (Pritchett and Seeburg 1990;

Table 2. Affinities of BZ ligands for $GABA_A$-receptor subtypes (from Lüddens et al. 1990; Pritchett and Seeburg 1990; Pritchett et al. 1989)

	$\alpha_1\beta_1\gamma_2$	$\alpha_2\beta_1\gamma_2$	$\alpha_3\beta_1\gamma_2$	$\alpha_5\beta_3\gamma_2$	$\alpha_4\beta_2\gamma_2$	$\alpha_6\beta_2\gamma_2$
Ro 15-1788	0.5 ± 0.2	1.2 ± 0.1	0.7 ± 0.2	0.5 ± 0.1	107 ± 26	90 ± 20
CL 218 872	130 ± 40	1790 ± 620	1500 ± 230	490 ± 120	$>10\,000$	$>10\,000$
2-oxoquazepam	20 ± 3	225 ± 12	201 ± 18	190 ± 15	$>10\,000$	$>10\,000$
Zolpidem	N.D.	450 ± 21	400 ± 43	$>10\,000$	N.D.	$>10\,000$
[^{3}H]ligand	Ro 15-1788	Ro 15-1788	Ro 15-1788	Ro 15-1788	Ro 15-4513	Ro 15-4513

Shown are the affinities of four BZ-receptor ligands in nM $\pm$ standard error of mean. The receptors were obtained by transient transfection of 293 human embryonic kidney cells with plasmid vectors coding for the listed rat $GABA_A$-receptor subunits. N.D., not determined.

Pritchett et al. 1989; Table 2). So far, no BZ-receptor ligand distinguishes between the $\alpha_2\beta_x\gamma_2$ and $\alpha_3\beta x\gamma_2$ receptors, but both display the characteristics of the "classical" BZ type II receptors described in the mammalian brain. Transiently expressed $\alpha_5\beta_2\gamma_2$ receptors have affinities for CL 218 872 and 2-oxoquazepam similar to α_2 or α_3 containing $\alpha_x\beta_x\gamma_2$ receptors (Table 2). However, the binding properties for imidazopyridines like zolpidem and alpidem differ from conventional $GABA_A$/BZ II receptors (Pritchett and Seeburg 1990), so they constitute a subtype of the BZ II receptors.

BZ I and BZ II receptors distribute unevenly over the rat brain. BZ I receptors predominate in the cerebellum, but are rare in the hippocampus (Faull and Villinger 1988; Faull et al. 1987; Olsen et al. 1990). On the other hand, BZ II receptors are strongly expressed in the hippocampus and nearly absent from the cerebellum, whereas both receptor subtypes are similarly expressed in the cortical layers (Faull and Villinger 1988; Faull et al. 1987; Olsen et al. 1990). Data derived from ligand binding to recombinant receptors are in good agreement with the mRNA distribution of the α subunits. Areas rich in BZ I receptors have high contents of the α_1 mRNA, and the sum of the α_2, α_3, and α_5 mRNA levels in the brain correlates with the pattern of the BZ II receptor type (Laurie et al. 1992; Wisden et al. 1992). On its own, the α_5 mRNA is highly enriched in CA1 and CA3 of the hippocampus, the granule cells of the olfactory bulb, and the entorhinal and infralimbic cortex (Laurie et al. 1992; Wisden et al. 1992), exactly those structures of the rat brain containing the highest levels of zolpidem-insensitive BZ II receptors. These data strongly indicate that transiently expressed $\alpha_1\beta_x\gamma_2$, $\alpha_2\beta_x\gamma_2$, $\alpha_3\beta_x\gamma_2$, or $\alpha_5\beta_2\gamma_2$ receptors reflect properties of their counterparts in the brain. This view is supported by the immunopurification of $GABA_AR$ subtypes solubilized from rat brain that display affinities comparable to those measured in transiently transfected cells (McKernan et al. 1991). It had previously been shown by sequential immunoprecipitation using antibodies specific for the α_1, α_2, and α_3 variants that iso-oligomers of the $GABA_AR$ exist in bovine brain (Duggan and Stephenson 1990).

3.2.2 Diazepam-Insensitive GABA$_A$/BZ Receptors

One of the α subunits, α_6, is restricted to cerebellar granule cells (Lüddens et al. 1990). The recombinant receptor expressing it in 293 cells, together with β_2 and γ_2, bind with high affinity the GABA agonist [^{3}H]muscimol and the imidazo-1, 4-benzodiazepine [^{3}H]Ro 15-4513. Other BZ and two β-carbolines were either not recognized by this receptor or at an affinity two to three orders of magnitude lower than that for α_1-, α_2-, α_3-, or α_5-containing receptors (Lüddens et al. 1990; Pritchett and Seeburg 1990; Pritchett et al. 1989).

In addition to the 50-kDa band corresponding to α_1, a band with an M_r of 57 kDa was revealed by autoradiography of [^{3}H]Ro 15-4513-photolabeled cerebellar membranes (Lüddens et al. 1990). However, only the incorporation of the [^{3}H]Ro 15-4513 photolabel into the 50-kDa band was inhibited by 10 μM diazepam (Lüddens et al. 1990) showing that a receptor with a pharmacology similar to the recombinant $\alpha_6\beta_2\gamma_2$ receptor is present in rat brain. Several, but not all BZ-receptor ligands displace all [^{3}H]Ro 15-4513 binding from cerebellar membranes. The affinities of these ligands correspond well with the data obtained from recombinant receptors: In two alcohol-tolerant and nontolerant rat lines (Uusi-Oukari and Korpi 1990), as well as in membranes derived from Sprague-Dawley rat, bovine, or human cerebellum (Lüddens et al. 1990; Turner et al. 1991; Wong and Skolnick 1992) inhibition of [^{3}H]Ro 15-4513 binding was best fitted to two-site curves in which the low-affinity site was present in relative abundance (20%–30%) and was made up most likely of α_6-containing receptors.

The cerebellar Ro 15 4513-selective GABA$_A$R subtype may well assemble from α_6, β_2, and γ_2 subunits, consistent with the simultaneous expression of these subunits in the cerebellar granule cells (Shivers et al. 1989; Wisden et al. 1988), although other subunit combinations with or without α_6 might result in a similar pharmacology. An initial functional evaluation of 293 cells expressing $\alpha_6\beta_2\gamma_2$ receptors indicated a decrease in the GABA-evoked current by the two inverse agonists Ro 15-4513 and DMCM, while variable effects of the full agonist flunitrazepam were observed (Kleingoor et al. 1991). Contrasting data were obtained using the GABA shift of BZ-binding data as a measure of the functionality of the GABA and BZ site coupling (Wong and Skolnick 1992). In this study it was concluded that the diazepam-insensitive sites recognize BZ, but that the BZ receptor has no functional coupling to the intrinsic channel pore of GABA$_A$R complex, i.e., that no BZ-receptor ligand so far modulates the GABA response of the diazepam-insensitive GABA$_A$ channels. However, at low concentrations of DMCM a small but significant GABA shift has been observed for the β-carboline DMCM (Turner et al. 1991).

By in vitro transfection of the β_2 and γ_2 subunits together with the α_4 variant, a receptor was created with pharmacological properties similar to those of $\alpha_6\beta_2\gamma_2$ receptors (Wisden et al. 1991). In contrast to the latter receptor, the in vivo existence of $\alpha_4\beta_2\gamma_2$ receptors in the brain awaits verification. It is already obvious (by the presence of α_4 mRNA in rat thalamus and the virtual absence of diazepam-insensitive [^{3}H]Ro 15-4513 sites in this brain area) that α_4 assembles at least in the thalamus with partners other than β_x and γ_2 (Wisden et al. 1991, 1992).

3.3 Development of GABA$_A$R Subtypes

Studies employing subtype-selective imidazopyridines to investigate the developmental regulation of different GABA$_A$R indicated a postnatal onset of GABA$_A$/BZ I receptor expression that is concurrent with a decline in the proportion of GABA$_A$/BZ II receptors (Bacon et al. 1991; Eichinger and Sieghart 1986; Garrett and Tabakoff 1985; Vitorica et al. 1990). A similar pattern has been observed for the hippocampal expression of the mRNAs coding for the α variants in situ (Killisch et al. 1991). Here the α_1 mRNA was undetectable before birth, low around postnatal day 6 (P6), and increased to significant levels in the adult hippocampus (Killisch et al. 1991; Wisden et al. 1992). Similarly, α_3 mRNA was undetectable before birth, peaked between P6 and P12, but declined to the low adult expression thereafter. In contrast, α_5 mRNA was consistently found in the embryonic and the adult hippocampal formation (Killisch et al. 1991; Wisden et al. 1992). These results were corroborated by an in vitro system of primary hippocampal cells cultured for various periods of time. In these cells the α_1 protein was detected by an α_1-variant-specific antibody only late after plating of the cells, whereas the α_3 and α_5 subunits were present at all culture stages (Killisch et al. 1991). These developmental studies together with the described pharmacology of the GABA$_A$Receptor argue for the virtual absence of zolpidem-sensitive sites in the perinatal rat hippocampus.

4 Conclusion and Perspectives

Multiple GABA$_A$R exist in the brain that show differential distribution and developmental patterns. Their regulation by BZ-receptor ligands differs dramatically with the α variant present in the complex, whereas the EC$_{50}$ for GABA does not seem to be affected accordingly (Sigel et al. 1992). Additional variation of the GABA$_A$R comes with the exchange of the γ subunits, though the actual bearing on the in vivo system has still to be resolved.

Parts of the putative binding site for BZ ligands have been identified (Pritchett and Seeburg 1991; Wieland et al. 1992), but it will still take considerable effort before the BZ-binding pocket has been analyzed in full. Only the first steps have been taken towards the identification of the domains involved in the binding of the neurotransmitter itself (Sigel et al.

1992). No clear idea exists regarding the stoichiometry of the single subunits.

Indeed, great progress has been made in the characterization of neurotransmitter receptor systems, but there are still a number of questions to be resolved.

References

Bacon E, de Barry J, Gombos G (1991) Differential ontogenesis of type I and II benzodiazepine receptors in mouse cerebellum. Brain Res Dev Brain Res 58:283–287

Bateson AN, Lasham A, Darlison MG (1991) γ-Aminobutyric acid$_A$ receptor heterogeneity is increased by alternative splicing of a novel β-subunit gene transcript. J Neurochem 56:1437–1440

Benke D, Mertens S, Trzeciak A, Gillessen D, Mohler H (1991) Identification and immunohistochemical mapping of GABA$_A$ receptor subtypes containing the δ subunit in rat brain. FEBS Lett 283:145–149

Betz H (1990) Ligand-gated ion channels in the brain: the amino acid receptor superfamily. Neuron 5:383–392

Corda MG, Giorgi O, Longoni B, Ongini E, Montaldo S, Biggio G (1988) Preferential affinity of 3H-2-oxo-quazepam for type I benzodiazepine recognition sites in the human brain. Life Sci 42:189–197

Cutting GR, Lu L, Ohara BF, Kasch LM, Montroserafizadeh C, Donovan DM, Shimada S, Antonarakis SE, Guggino WB, Uhl GR, Kazazian HH (1991) Cloning of the γ-aminobutyric acid (GABA) ρ1 cDNA – A GABA receptor subunit highly expressed in the retina. Proc Natl Acad Sci USA 88:2673–2677

Dingledine R, Boland LM, Chamberlin NL, Kawasaki K, Kleckner NW, Traynelis SF, Verdoorn TA (1988) Amino acid receptors and uptake systems in the mammalian central nervous system. Crit Rev Neurobiol 4:1–96

Duggan MJ, Stephenson FA (1990) Biochemical evidence for the existence of γ-aminobutyrate$_A$ receptor iso-oligomers. J Biol Chem 265:3831–3835

Eichinger A, Sieghart W (1985) Differential degradation of different benzodiazepinebinding proteins by incubation of membranes from cerebellum or hippocampus with trypsin. J Neurochem 45:219–226

Eichinger A, Sieghart W (1986) Postnatal development of proteins associated with different benzodiazepine receptors. J Neurochem 46:173–180

Faull RL, Villiger JW (1988) Benzodiazepine receptors in the human hippocampal formation: a pharmacological and quantitative autoradiographic study. Neuroscience 26:783–790

Faull RL, Villiger JW, Holford NH (1987) Benzodiazepine receptors in the human cerebellar cortex: a quantitative autoradiographic and pharmacological study demonstrating the predominance of type I receptors. Brain Res 411:379–385

Garrett KM, Tabakoff B (1985) The development of type I and type II benzodiazepine receptors in the mouse cortex and cerebellum. Pharmacol Biochem Behav 22:985–992

Hebebrand J, Friedl W, Unverzagt B, Propping P (1986) Benzodiazepine receptor subunits in avian brain. J Neurochem 47:790–793

Herb A, Wisden W, Lüddens H, Puia G, Vicini S, Seeburg PH (1992) The third γ subunit of the γ-aminobutyric acid type A receptor family. Proc Natl Acad Sci USA 89:1433–1437

Kao PN, Karlin A (1986) Acetylcholine receptor-binding site contains a disulfide crosslink between adjacent half-cystinyl residues. J Biol Chem 261:8085–8088

Khrestchatisky M, MacLennan AJ, Chiang MY, Xu WT, Jackson MB, Brecha N, Sternini C, Olsen RW, Tobin AJ (1989) A novel α subunit in rat brain $GABA_A$ receptors. Neuron 3:745–753

Killisch I, Dotti CG, Laurie DJ, Lüddens H, Seeburg H (1991) Expression patterns of $GABA_A$ receptor subtypes in developing hippocampal neurons. Neuron 7:927–936

Kleingoor C, Ewert M, Von Blankenfeld G, Seeburg PH, Kettenmann H (1991) Inverse but not full benzodiazepine agonists modulate recombinant $α_6β_2γ_2$ $GABA_A$ receptors in transfected human embryonic kidney cells. Neurosci Lett 130:169–172

Knoflach F, Rhyner T, Villa M, Kellenberger S, Drescher U, Malherbe P, Sigel E, Mohler H (1991) The $γ_3$ subunit of the $GABA_A$ receptor confers sensitivity to benzodiazepine-receptor ligands. FEBS Lett 293:191–194

Kofuji P, Wang JB, Moss SJ, Huganir RL, Burt DR (1991) Generation of two forms of the γ-aminobutyric acid$_A$ receptor $γ_2$ subunit in mice by alternative splicing. J Neurochem 56:713–715

Laurie DJ, Seeburg PH, Wisden W (1992) The distribution of 13 $GABA_A$ receptor subunit mRNAs in the rat brain. II. Olfactory Bulb and Cerebellum. J Neurosci 12:1063–1076

Levitan ES, Schofield PR, Burt DR, Rhee LM, Wisden W, Köhler M, Fujita N, Rodriguez HF, Stephenson FA, Darlison MG, Barnard E, Seeburg PH (1988) Structural and functional basis for $GABA_A$ receptor heterogeneity. Nature 335:76–79

Lo MM, Niehoff DL, Kuhar MJ, Snyder SH (1983) Differential localization of type I and type II benzodiazepine-binding sites in substantia nigra. Nature 306:57–60

Lüddens H, Pritchett DB, Köhler M, Killisch I, Keinänen K, Monyer H, Sprengel R, Seeburg PH (1990) Cerebellar $GABA_A$ receptor selective for a behavioural alcohol antagonist. Nature 346:648–651

Lüddens H, Wisden W (1991) Function and pharmacology of multiple $GABA_A$ receptor subunits. Trends Pharmacol Sci 12:49–51

Lueddens HW, Skolnick P (1987) "Peripheral-type" benzodiazepine receptors in the kidney: regulation of radioligand binding by anions and DIDS. Eur J Pharmacol 133:205–214

Malherbe P, Draguhn A, Multhaup G, Beyreuther K, Möhler H (1990a) $GABA_A$ receptor expressed from rat brain α- and β-subunit cDNAs displays potentiation by benzodiazepine-receptor ligands. Brain Res Mol Brain Res 8:199–208

Malherbe P, Sigel E, Baur R, Persohn E, Richards JG, Möhler H (1990b) Functional characteristics and sites of gene expression of the $α_1$, $β_1$, $γ_2$-isoform of the rat $GABA_A$ receptor. J Neurosci 10:2330–2337

Maricq AV, Peterson AS, Brake AJ, Myers RM, Julius D (1991) Primary structure and functional expression of the $5HT_3$ receptor, a serotonin-gated ion channel. Science 254:432–437

McKernan RM, Quirk K, Prince R, Cox PA, Gillard NP, Ragan CI, Whiting P (1991) $GABA_A$ receptor subtypes immunopurified from rat brain with subunit-specific antibodies have unique pharmacological properties. Neuron 7:667–676

Monyer H, Sprengel R, Schoepfer R, Herb A, Higuchi M, Lomeli H, Burnashev N, Sakmann B, Seeburg PH (1992) Heteromeric NMDA receptors: molecular and functional distinction of subtypes. Science 256:1217–1221

Moriyoshi K, Masu M, Ishii T, Shigemoto R, Mizuno N, Nakanishi S (1991) Molecular cloning and characterization of the rat NMDA receptor. Nature 354:31–37

Mosckovitz R, Gershoni JM (1988) Three possible disulfides in the acetylcholine receptor alpha subunit. J Biol Chem 263:1017–1022

Nielsen M, Braestrup C (1980) Ethyl β-carboline-3-carboxylate shows differential benzodiazepine-receptor interaction. Nature 286:606–607

Olsen RW, McCabe RT, Wamsley JK (1990) $GABA_A$ receptor subtypes: autoradiographic comparison of GABA, benzodiazepine, and convulsant-binding sites in the rat central nervous system. J Chem Neuroanat 3:59–76

Olsen RW, Tobin AJ (1990) Molecular biology of $GABA_A$ receptors. FASEB J 4:1469–1480

Pritchett DB, Lüddens H, Seeburg PH (1989) Type I and type II GABA$_A$-benzodiaze-pine receptors produced in transfected cells. Science 245:1389–1392

Pritchett DB, Seeburg PH (1990) γ-Aminobutyric acid$_A$ receptor α$_5$ subunit creates novel type II benzodiazepine-receptor pharmacology. J Neurochem 54:1802–1804

Pritchett DB, Seeburg PH (1991) γ-Aminobutyric acid type A receptor point mutation increases the affinity of compounds for the benzodiazepine site. Proc Natl Acad Sci USA 88:1421–1425

Pritchett DB, Sontheimer H, Shivers BD, Ymer S, Kettenmann H, Schofield PR, See-burg PH (1989) Importance of a novel GABA$_A$-receptor subunit for benzodiazepine pharmacology. Nature 338:582–585

Schofield PR, Darlison MG, Fujita N, Burt DR, Stephenson FA, Rodriguez H, Rhee LM, Ramachandran J, Reale V, Glencorse TA, Reale V, Seeburg PH, Barnard EA (1987) Sequence and functional expression of the GABA$_A$ receptor shows a ligand-gated receptor super-family. Nature 328:221–227

Seeburg PH, Wisden W, Verdoorn TA, Pritchett DB, Werner P, Herb A, Lüddens H, Sprengel R, Sakmann B (1990) The GABA$_A$ receptor family: molecular and func-tional diversity. CSH Symp Quant Biol 55:29–44

Sequier JM, Richards JG, Malherbe P, Price GW, Mathews S, Möhler H (1988) Mapping of brain areas containing RNA homologous to cDNAs encoding the α and β sub-units of the rat GABA$_A$ γ-aminobutyrate receptor. Proc Natl Acad Sci USA 85: 7815–7819

Shimada S, Cutting GR, Uhl GR (1992) γ-Aminobutyric acid A or C receptor? γ-Aminobutyric acid ρ$_1$ receptor RNA induces bicuculline-, barbiturate-, and benzo-diazepine-insensitive γ-aminobutyric acid responses in *Xenopus* oocytes. Mol Phar-macol 41:683–687

Shivers BD, Killisch I, Sprengel R, Sontheimer H, Köhler M, Schofield PR, Seeburg PH (1989) Two novel GABA$_A$ receptor subunits exist in distinct neuronal subpopula-tions. Neuron 3:327–337

Sieghart W (1983) Several new banzodiazepines selectively interact with a benzodiazepine receptor subtype. Neurosci Lett 38:73–78

Sieghart W, Eichinger A, Riederer P, Jellinger K (1985) Comparison of benzodiazepine-receptor binding in membranes from human or rat brain. Neuropharmacology 24:751–759

Sieghart W, Karobath M (1980) Molecular heterogeneity of benzodiazepine receptors. Nature 286:285–287

Sigel E, Baur R, Kellenberger S, Malherbe P (1992) Point mutations affecting antago-nist affinity and agonist-dependent gating of GABA$_A$ receptor channels. EMBO J 11:2017–2023

Sigel E, Baur R, Trube G, Möhler H, Malherbe P (1990) The effect of subunit composi-tion of rat brain GABA$_A$ receptors on channel function. Neuron 5:703–711

Sigel E, Stephenson FA, Mamalaki C, Barnard EA (1983) A γ-aminobutyric acid/benzo-diazepine-receptor complex of bovine cerebral cortex. J Biol Chem 258:6965–6971

Squires RF, Benson DI, Braestrup C, Coupet J, Klepner CA, Myers V, Beer B (1979) Some properties of brain-specific benzodiazepine receptors: new evidence for mul-tiple receptors. Pharmacol Biochem Behav 10:825–830

Turner DM, Sapp DW, Olsen RW (1991) The benzodiazepine/alcohol antagonist Ro-15-24513 – binding to a GABA$_A$ receptor subtype that is insensitive to diazepam. J Pharmacol Exp Ther 257:1236–1242

Unwin N (1989) The structure of ion channels in membranes of excitable cells. Neuron 3:665–676

Uusi-Oukari M, Korpi ER (1990) Diazepam sensitivity of an imidazobenzodiazepine, [^{3}H]Ro 15-4513, in cerebellar membranes from two rat lines developed for high and low alcohol sensitivity. J Neurochem 54:1980–1987

Vitorica J, Park D, Chin G, de Blas A (1990) Characterization with antibodies of the γ-aminobutyric acid$_A$/benzodiazepine-receptor complex during development of the rat brain. J Neurochem 54:187–194

Wafford KA, Burnett DM, Leidenheimer NJ, Burt DR, Wang JB, Kofuji P, Dunwiddie TV, Harris RA, Sikela JM (1991) Ethanol sensitivity of the GABA$_A$ receptor expressed in *Xenopus* oocytes requires eight amino acids contained in the gamma 2L subunit. Neuron 7:27–33

Whiting PW, McKernan RM, Iversen LL (1990) Another mechanism for generating GABA$_A$-receptor heterogeneity: alternative splicing of the γ_2 subunit generates two forms, one of which contains a consensus sequence for protein kinase C. Proc Natl Acad Sci USA 87:9966–9970

Wieland H, Lüddens H, Seeburg PH (1992) A single histidine in GABA$_A$ receptors is essential for benzodiazepine-agonist binding. J Biol Chem 257:1426–1429

Wisden W, Herb A, Wieland H, Keinänen K, Lüddens H, Seeburg PH (1991) Cloning, pharmacological characteristics, and expression pattern of the rat GABA$_A$ receptor α_4 subunit. FEBS Lett 289:227–230

Wisden W, Laurie DJ, Monyer H, Seeburg PH (1992) The distribution of 13 GABA$_A$-receptor subunit mRNAs in the rat brain. I. Telencephalon, Diencephalon, Mesencephalon. J Neurosci 12:1040–1062

Wisden W, Morris BJ, Darlison MG, Hunt SP, Barnard EA (1988) Distinct GABA$_A$ receptor α subunit mRNAs show differential patterns of expression in bovine brain. Neuron 1:937–947

Wong G, Skolnick P (1992) High affinity ligands for "diazepam-insensitive" benzodiazepine receptors. Eur J Pharmacol 225:63–68

Ymer S, Draguhn A, Köhler M, Seeburg PH (1989a) Sequence and expression of a novel GABA$_A$ receptor α subunit. FEBS Lett 258:119–122

Ymer S, Schofield PR, Draguhn A, Werner P, Köhler M, Seeburg PH (1989b) GABA$_A$-receptor β-subunit heterogeneity: functional expression of cloned cDNAs. EMBO J 8:1665–1670

Ymer S, Draguhn A, Wisden W, Werner P, Keinänen K, Schofield PR, Sprengel R, Pritchett DB, Seeburg PH (1990) Structural and functional characterization of the γ_1 subunit of GABA$_A$/benzodiazepine receptors. EMBO J 9:3261–3267

Zimprich F, Zezula J, Sieghart W, Lassmann H (1991) Immunohistochemical localization of the α_1, α_2, and α_3 subunit of the GABA$_A$ receptor in the rat brain. Neurosci Lett 127:125–128

Immunohistochemical Mapping of Gamma-Aminobutyric Acid Type-A Receptor Alpha Subunits in Rat Central Nervous System

J.D. Turner[1], G. Bodewitz[1], C.L. Thompson[2], and F.A. Stephenson[2]

1 Introduction

The inhibitory γ-aminobutyric acid type A ($GABA_A$) receptors of mammalian brain are hetero-oligomeric membrane glycoproteins, in which five subunits are thought to assemble to form individual chloride-channel complexes bearing $GABA_A$ receptors and their associated modulatory sites. Five distinct subunit classes, some containing several isoforms (α_{1-6}, β_{1-3}, γ_{1-3}, δ and ρ_{1-2}) encoded by separate genes, have been identified by molecular cloning (see e.g., Olsen and Tobin 1990; Stephenson 1991). Recombinant receptors assembled from these subunits possess heterogeneous pharmacological and biophysical properties, with the pharmacological properties of the principal allosteric modulatory site (the benzodiazepine receptor, BZR) being determined by the α and/or γ species present (see e.g., Lüddens and Wisden 1991). The combinations which assemble in vivo to constitute native receptors are not known, but in situ hybridisation studies have demonstrated not only overlapping but also distinct distributions of the mRNAs coding for the different subunit classes and isoforms (e.g., Laurie et al. 1992; Wisden et al. 1992). While ligand-binding studies in brain membranes employing compounds such as zolpidem (Niddam et al. 1987) have previously provided evidence for the existence of two classes of BZR (termed BZ1 and BZ2 or $\omega1$ and $\omega2$), this recent evidence from molecular biological studies suggests the presence of subclasses at least of the BZ2 type (e.g., Pritchett and Seeburg 1990).

To facilitate biochemical isolation and identification of putative subtypes of native GABA receptors, and for characterisation of their function, it is necessary to obtain information about the relative distributions of the different subunits. In addition, this information is important for the interpretation of the pharmacological profiles of compounds such as abecarnil, which show selectivity for certain recombinant receptor subtypes (see Pribilla et al., this volume). While in situ hybridisation studies can demonstrate the distribution of mRNAs, this need not coincide with the distribution of the

[1] Research Laboratories of Schering AG, Berlin 65, Germany
[2] School of Pharmacy, University of London, London, UK

protein products if they are targetted to anatomically specific locations on cell membranes, and they give no direct information about the constitution of individual receptors. We have therefore raised antibodies to peptide sequences unique to the α_1, α_2, α_3, α_5 and α_6 subunits of the GABA$_A$ receptor and have used these to map the distributions of these subunits in rat brain.

2 Mapping with Immunohistochemistry: α Subunits Have Unique Distributions

Polyclonal antibodies were raised in rabbits to the following synthetic peptide sequences which are unique to the respective subunits: PEKPK-KVKDPLIKKNNT (α_1 322–338, rat), CLNREPVLGVSP (Cys-α_2 414–424, rat), CVNRESAIKGMIRKQ (Cys-α_3 454–467, rat), QMPTSSVQDET-NDNITC (α_5 1–16-Cys, rat) and KLEDEGNFYSKNISRIL (α_6 1–17, bovine) coupled to keyhole-limpet haemocyanin (for sequences see Pritchett and Seeburg 1990 and Lüddens et al. 1990). Antisera were affinity purified using the respective peptide-affinity columns (Duggan and Stephenson 1990). Conventional immunohistochemical procedures were employed, using free-floating paraformaldehyde-fixed sections of adult rat brain, antibody concentrations ranging from 0.025–4 µg/ml and detection using peroxidase–antiperoxidase. Specificity controls were carried out by adsorption of primary antibodies at working dilutions with their respective peptides (1–2 µg/ml) prior to application to the tissue. In all cases this step abolished either all, or a major part of the staining elicited by untreated antibody.

2.1 Global Distribution of α Subunits

The different antibodies elicited characteristic, specific staining patterns throughout the central nervous system (CNS; Fig. 1 and Table 1). The patterns overlapped in many brain areas (e.g., cortex, olfactory bulb) but were mutually exclusive in others (e.g., basal forebrain, substantia nigra). The most abundant and widely distributed were α_{1-3}-like immunoreactivities (LIR), while α_5- and α_6-LIR were, respectively, much more restricted. Inspection of the distributions of the different subunit LIR reveals a good but incomplete match with the distribution patterns of the respective mRNAs (see Laurie et al. 1992; Wisden et al. 1992). The most significant mismatch was observed for α_3 in striatum and thalamus (see below for discussion).

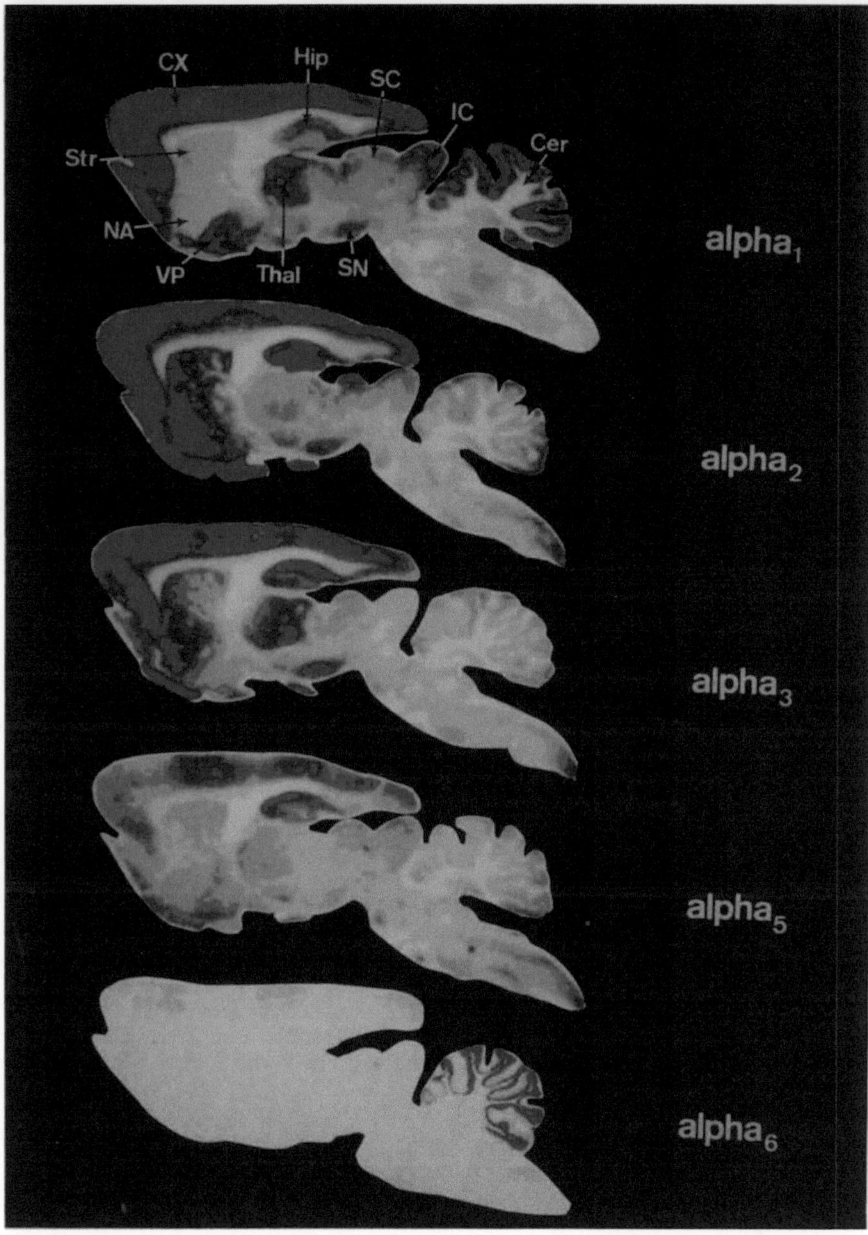

Fig. 1. Global distributions in rat brain of alpha-subunit immunoreactivity. Image analysis of sagittal sections stained with each of the antibodies reveals the sites of most abundant immunoreaction (red > grey > white). Note that the patterns are complementary in many brain regions

Table 1. Distribution of GABA-receptor α-subunit-LIR in rat CNS

	α_1	α_2	α_3	α_5	α_6
Cortex	+++	++	+++	(+)	−
Hippocampus					
DG	+	+++	+	(+)	−
CA1	+	+++	++	+	−
CA3	+	+++	+	++	−
Interneurons	+++	−	(+)	−	−
Striatum	(+)	++	++	(+)	−
Acc.	−	++	+	−	−
OT	−	++	+	−	−
Pallidum	+++	+	+	(+)	−
Entoped.	+++	−	(+)	−	−
Septal nuclei	+++	+	+	(+)	−
Thalamus	+++	(+)	+++	(+)	−
Amygdala	++	++	++	−	−
Hypothalamus	+	+	+	(+)	−
SN	+++	(+)	++	(+)	−
Collic. sup.	+	+++	+	(+)	−
Collic. inf.	+++	(+)	+	(+)	−
Cerebellum					
ML	+++	++	(+)	(+)	−
PC	+++	++	(+)	++	−
GL	+++	−	(+)	(+)	+++
Brain stem	(+)	(+)	(+)	(+)	−
Spinal cord					
Dorsal	(+)	(+)	++	(+)	−
Ventral		+++	(+)	(+)	
Olfactory Bulb					
Glom.	++	(+)	+	+++	−
EPL	+++	(+)	+++	(+)	
Mitrals	+++	(+)	(+)	−	−
GL	(+)	(+)	(+)	++	−

Qualitative assessment of the relative distributions of alpha subunits demonstrated by immunocytochemistry.

+, ++, +++, increasing intensity of specific cellular or process staining; (+), only scattered cell bodies or processes; −, no staining; Acc., nucleus accumbens; DG, dentate gyrus; Entoped., entopeduncular nucleus; EPL, external plexiform layer; GL, granular layer; ML, molecular layer; OT, olfactory tubercle; PC, Purkinje cells; SN, substantia nigra.

2.2 Comparison of the Distributions of α Subunits in Different Brain Areas

2.2.1 Neocortex

The most abundant species were α_1-, α_2- and α_3-LIR and each showed a characteristic laminar distribution which was largely maintained throughout the cortex. As shown in Fig. 2 in frontal sections of temporal cortex, highest staining density with the α_1 antiserum was associated with layer IV. This

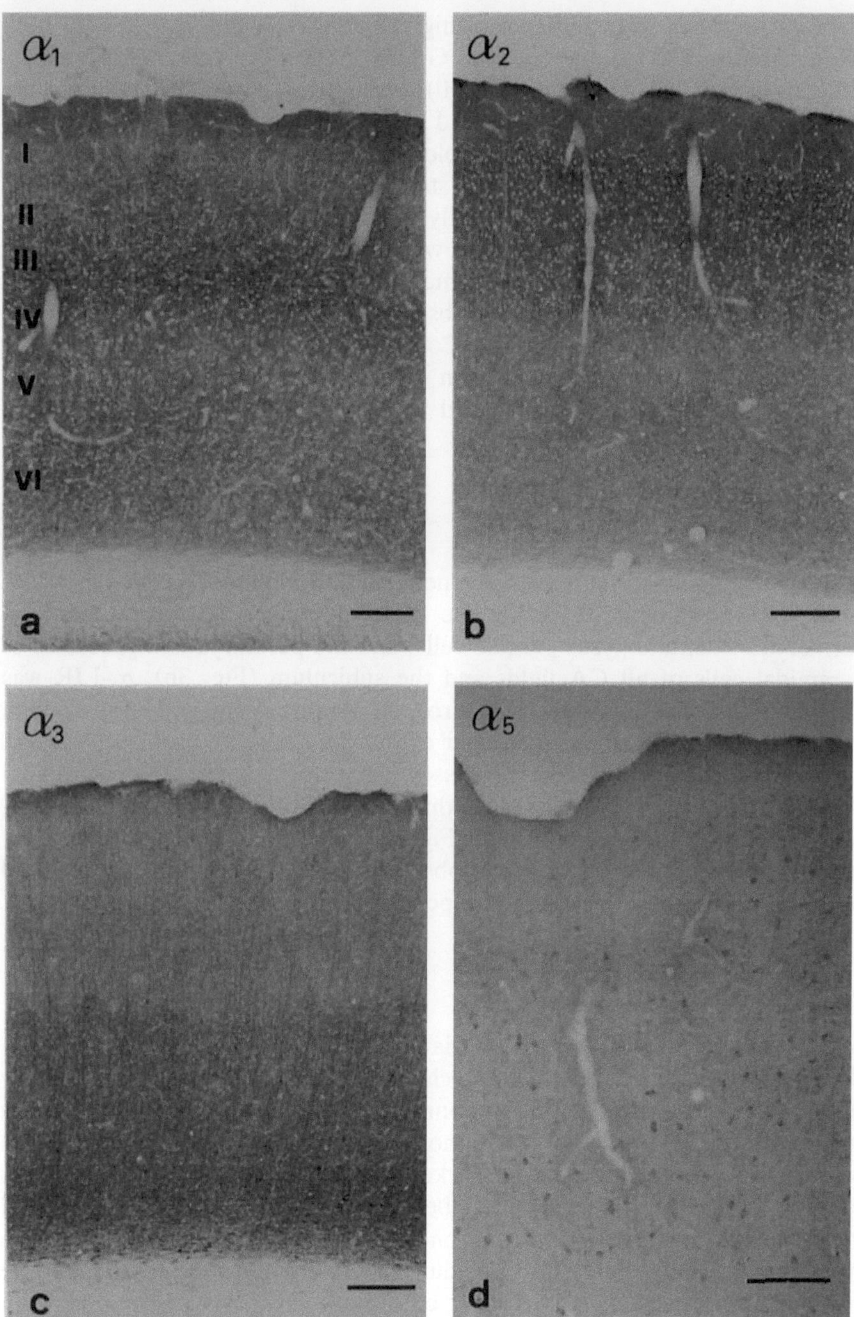

Fig. 2a–d. The most abundant species, α_1, α_2 and α_3 display similar laminar distributions throughout the cerebral cortex. In frontal sections of occipital cortex the complementary, but overlapping patterns of immunoreactivity are evident. Note how the highest α_1 density occurs in layers III–IV (**a**), while α_2 (**b**) and α_3 (**c**) are concentrated in layers I–III and V–VI, respectively, (**d**) α_5-LIR is associated with interneurones. *Scale bars* represent 200 μm

layer corresponds with the layer of highest density of binding sites for both BZR ligands and ligands for the $GABA_A$ receptor (own observations; Niddam et al. 1987; Olsen et al. 1990). In contrast, α_2 and α_3 staining were most concentrated in layers I–III and V–VI, respectively (Fig. 2a–c).

In sections of the thickness employed here, viewed in the optical microscope, it is difficult to identify the stained elements (i.e., dendrites, axons or even neuronal perikarya) especially when the intensity of staining is very high. However, α_1 and α_2 staining was of a very fine particulate quality suggesting that it was widely distributed on processes in the neuropile, and additional cellular profiles could be observed. In contrast, α_3-immunoreactive profiles were considerably coarser. Consistent staining with the α_5 antibody was seen only in a small population of presumed interneurones scattered throughout the cortex (Fig. 2d) and with some pyramidal cells in frontal cortex (Thompson et al. 1992).

2.2.2 Hippocampal Formation

In the hippocampus, the most prominent subunit immunoreactivity was that of α_2, which stained principally the molecular layer dendritic fields and perikarya of dentate gyrus granule cells, and the perikarya and processes of pyramidal cells of all CA fields and the subiculum (Fig. 3b). α_1-LIR was associated principally with interneurones, staining heavily their perikarya and processes and stained to a lesser extent the dendritic processes of CA1 pyramids (Fig. 3a). Coarse processes, concentrated in CA1 pyramidal dendritic fields and in the internal third of dentate gyrus molecular layer, were labelled by the α_3 antibody (Fig. 3c). The most conspicuous α_5-like staining in the entire forebrain was observed in the hippocampus, associated principally with the CA3 pyramidal perikarya (Fig. 3d).

2.2.3 Basal Ganglia

Most prominent staining in the striatum was obtained with the antibody directed against the α_2 peptide, which labelled heavily and homogeneously in the adult rat throughout striatum, nucleus accumbens and olfactory tubercle (e.g., Fig. 4b), but was almost undetectable in the globus pallidus and entopeduncular nucleus. In marked contrast, α_1-LIR was hardly detectable in the striatum, nucleus accumbens and olfactory tubercle, but stained very heavily large multipolar neurones and their processes in the globus pallidus, especially the ventral pallidum (Fig. 4a,d–f), and also stained the entopeduncular nucleus (the rodent equivalent of the internal pallidum in primates and man). α_3-LIR was associated with fine processes in the dorsal striatum and olfactory tubercle, and to a lesser extent the nucleus accumbens, and the antibody stained lightly cell bodies in the ventral pallidum and entopeduncular nucleus (Fig. 4c).

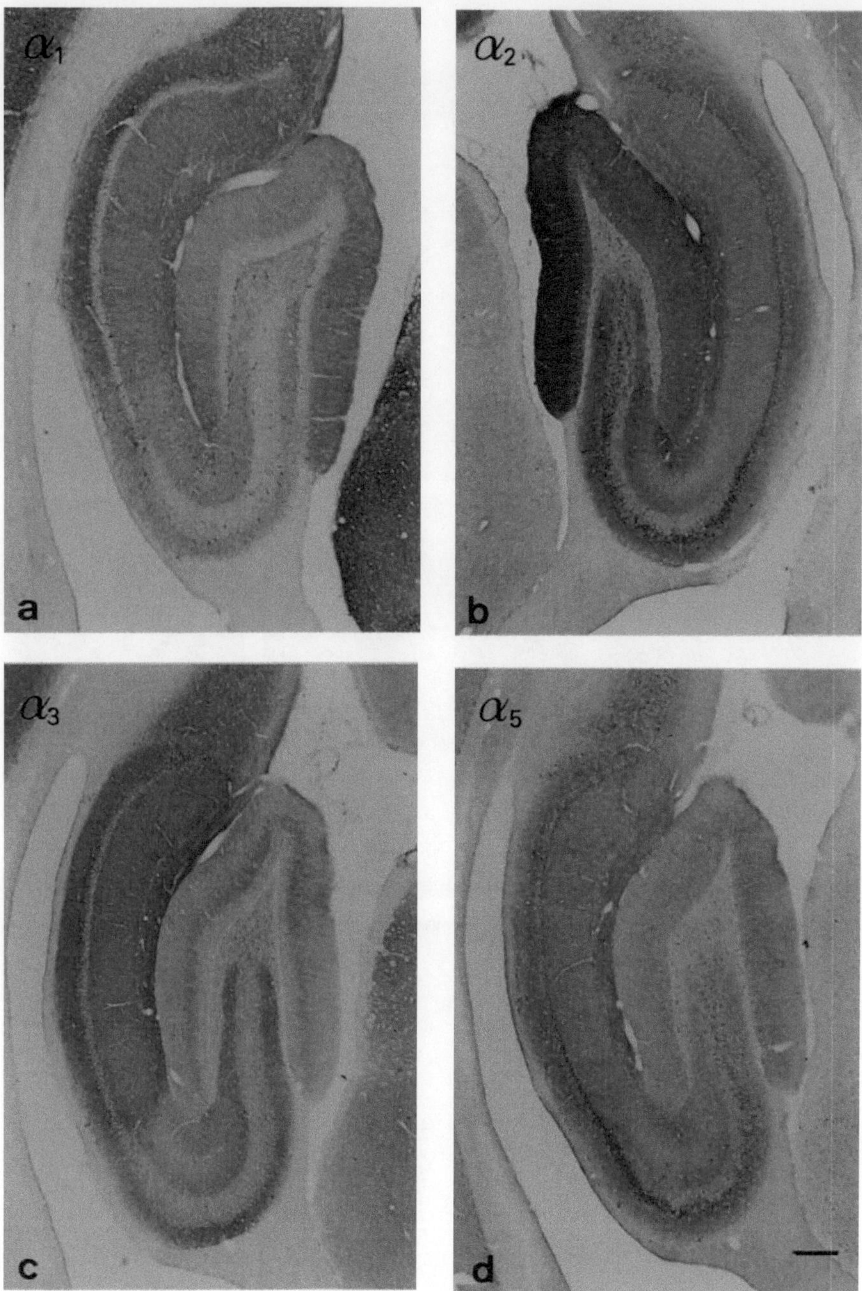

Fig. 3a–d. Characteristic immunoreactivity patterns are observed in the hippocampus, where **a** α_1-LIR decorates principally interneurones and to a lesser extent presumed pyramidal cell dendrites, mostly in the CA1 field. **b** In contrast, α_2-LIR is most prominent in the molecular layer of the dentate gyrus, and on the somata of granule and pyramidal, especially CA3, cells. **c** α_3-LIR appears most concentrated in the stratum oriens of all pyramidal fields, and in the stratum radiatum of CA1 (note also the graded staining in dentate molecular layer). **d** Some of the most dense α_5-LIR is associated with pyramidal somata, particularly in CA3. *Scale bar* represents 200 µm

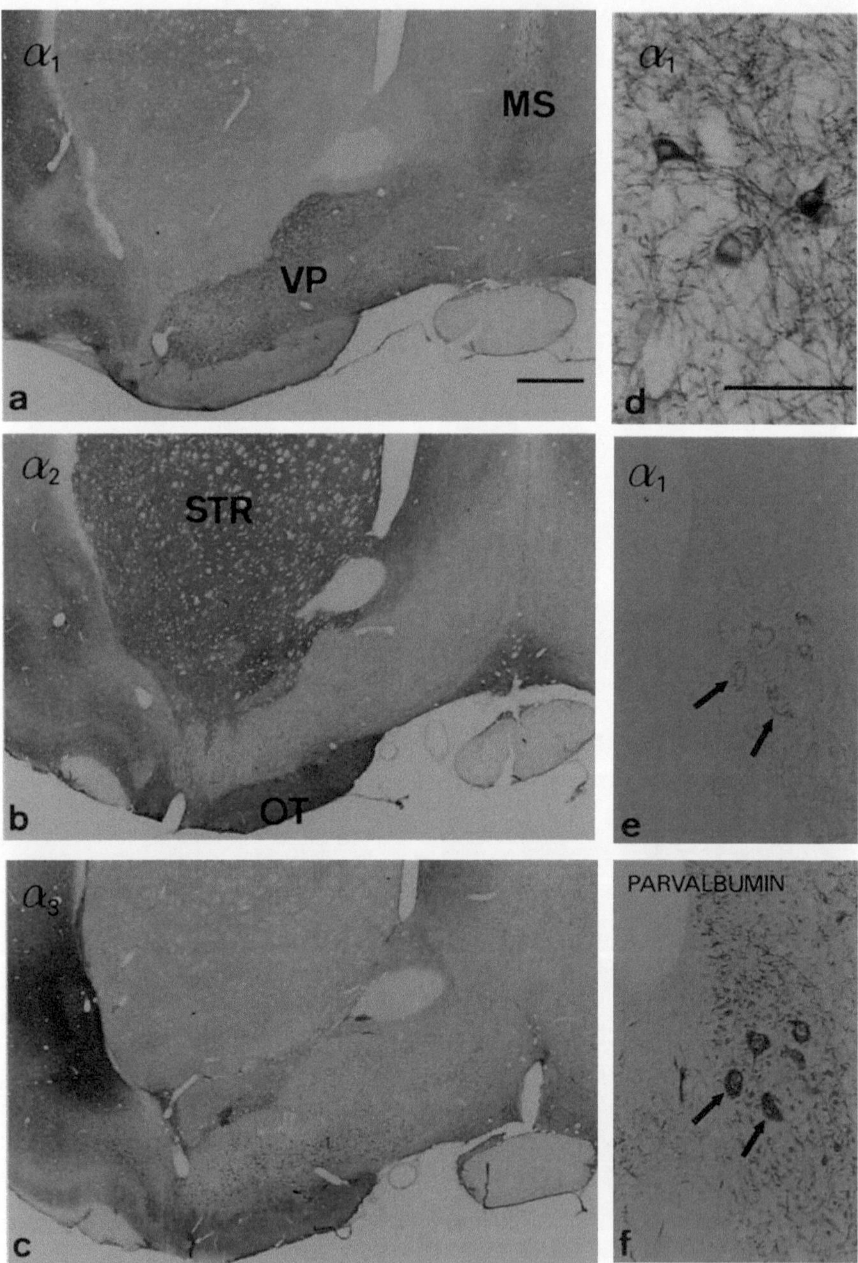

Fig. 4a–f. Striatum, basal forebrain and septum. **a** α_1-LIR is abundant in the basal forebrain, associated with large neurones and coarse processes (**d**) in the medial septum (*MS*) and ventral pallidum (*VP*). These neurones stain in consecutive thin sections for both α_1 and parvalbumin, a marker for GABAergic neurones (e.g., *arrows* in **e,f**). **b** A complementary pattern is revealed by the α_2 antiserum, which stains prominently but diffusely the striatum (*STR*) and the olfactory tubercle (*OT*). **c** Neuronal somata throughout the septal–pallidal complex contain α_3-LIR, but none of the α_1-positive processes appear labelled. *Scale bars* represent 500 μm (**a–c**) and 100 μm (**d–f**)

2.2.4 Septal Nuclei and Amygdala

Heterogeneous distributions of immunoreactivities for the different α subunits were evident in the septal nuclei where most prominent α_1 staining was associated with a subset of the hippocampally projecting medial septal neurones (Fig. 4a), while α_2 and α_3 were principally associated with neuronal cell bodies and processes in the lateral septum, in the dorsal and intermediate parts, respectively. Neurones in this part of the septal complex project onto medial septal neurones, forming part of the septo–hippocampo –septal loop system, which exerts a powerful influence on hippocampal activity and function (see Gray 1982). The α_1-containing neurones stained also for parvalbumin (Fig. 4e,f), an exclusive marker for GABAergic neurones in this brain area (Kiss et al. 1990). Strong α_1-LIR was seen on presumptive GABAergic neurones also in the substantia nigra, and many of the neurones in hippocampus, cortex and amygdala which showed α_1-LIR have morphologies typical of GABAergic interneurones or projection neurones. Staining of a separate population of medial septal neurones by the α_3 antiserum was also observed (e.g., Fig. 4c) and has been reported by others (e.g., Gao et al. 1992). Because a major proportion of large neurones in the medial septum and basal forebrain are cholinergic, attempts were made to colocalise α_3 and choline acetyl transferase (the synthetic enzyme for acetyl choline) in these neurones in sequential thin sections. Although these were unsuccessful, association of α_3-LIR with cholinergic neurones in this region has been reported by others (Gao et al. 1992). Likewise in the amygdala the different antibodies demonstrated contrasting staining patterns with α_1 being most concentrated, principally on fine processes but also on the perikarya of presumptive interneurones in the lateral nucleus, while α_2- and α_3-LIR were most prominent on fine processes in the central and basolateral nuclei, respectively (Fig. 5).

2.2.5 Thalamus

As seen in Fig. 1, the distributions of α_1 and α_3 subunits in thalamus were largely complementary, with α_1 more prominent in anterodorsal thalamus and α_3 more prominent in caudoventral regions. The two overlapped substantially, however, particularly in lateral posterior, dorsolateral geniculate and medial geniculate nuclei (e.g., Fig. 6a,b). While the distribution of α_1 staining can be predicted from in situ hybridisation demonstration of its mRNA, that of α_3 was quite unlike that of its mRNA, which is restricted to some midline nuclei and to the reticular nucleus of the thalamus (e.g., Wisden et al. 1992). Viewed at higher magnification, however, the α_3 staining appeared to be associated with profiles which could be the preterminal axonal processes of afferent inputs (Fig. 6c,d). Because the neurones of the reticular nucleus project heavily onto those nuclei which contain α_3-positive profiles, it is conceivable that the labelled processes emanate from them (because they contain α_3 mRNA and also stain lightly for α_3-LIR), and thus

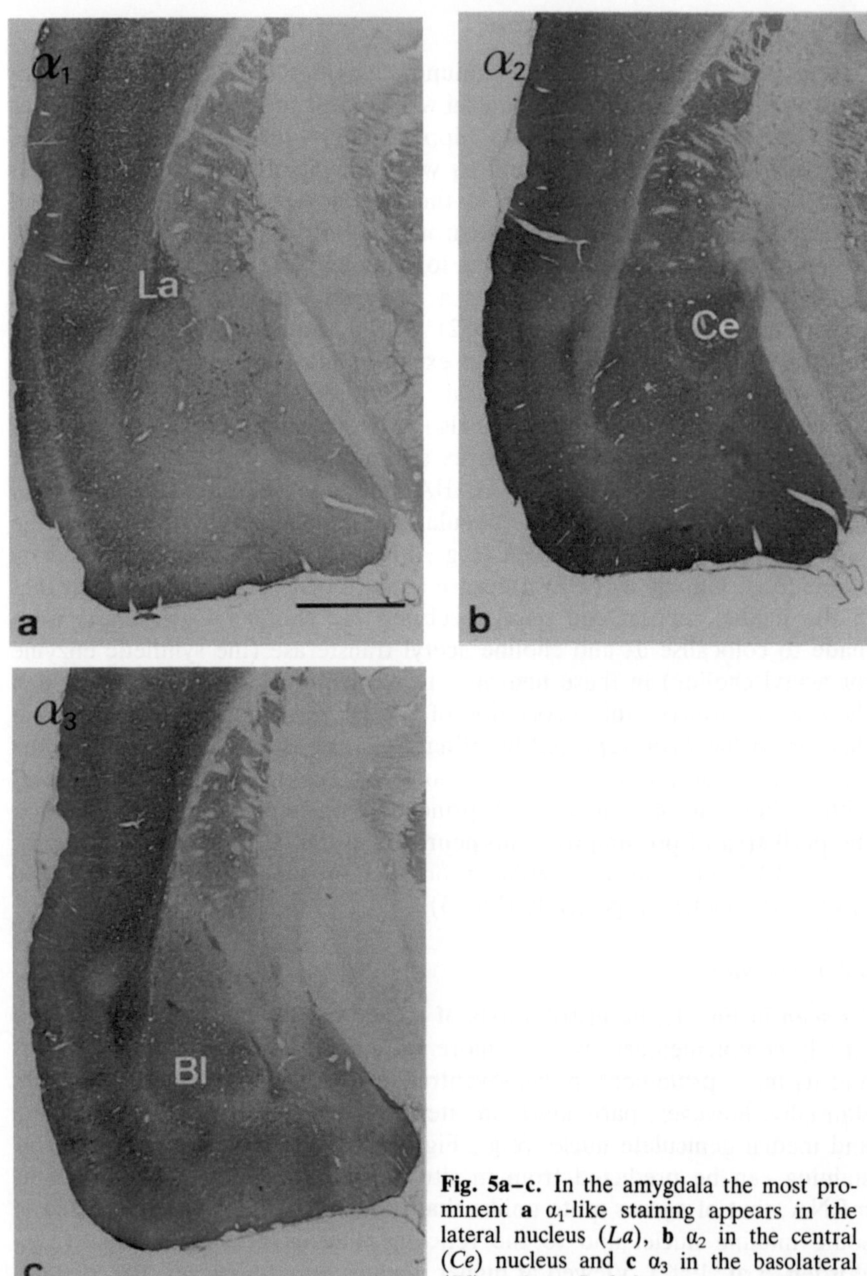

Fig. 5a–c. In the amygdala the most prominent **a** α_1-like staining appears in the lateral nucleus (*La*), **b** α_2 in the central (*Ce*) nucleus and **c** α_3 in the basolateral (*Bl*) nucleus. *Scale bar* represents 500 μm

Fig. 6a–d. Thalamus. In these sagittal sections, **a** α_1-LIR is most concentrated in dorsal nuclei (e.g., laterodorsal, *LD*, and posterolateral, *LP*) and is associated with zona incerta (*ZI*), subthalamic nucleus (*STN*) and with substantia nigra, pars reticulata (*SNR*) where coarse processes are labelled, while **b** α_3-LIR is prominent in more ventral

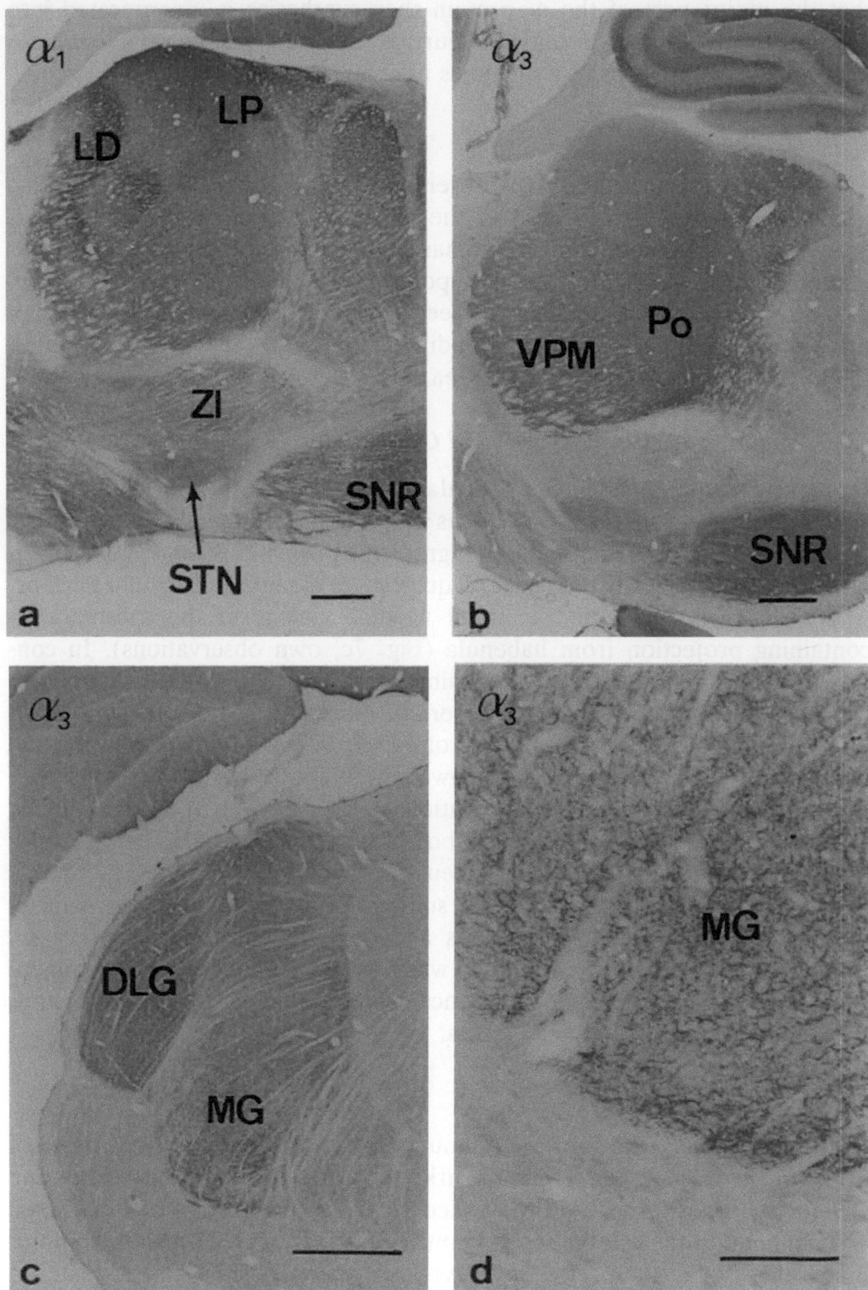

Fig. 6 (*contd.*)
structures (e.g., ventral posteriomedial, *VPM*, and posterior nuclei, *Po*), and label fine processes in *SNR*. **c** In frontal sections, α₃-staining is seen in the dorsolateral (*DLG*) and medial geniculate nuclei (*MG*) apparently on axonal or dendritic processes. **d** *Scale bars* represent 500 μm (**a–c**) and 100 μm (**d**)

that the major part of the α_3 protein they synthesise is incorporated into presynaptically located receptors. Further electron microscopic immuno-histochemical studies or lesion studies may help elucidate this.

2.2.6 Hypothalamus

The most abundant subunit-LIR observed in hypothalamus was that of α_2, which was present in neurones of the magnocellular neurones of the paraventricular, supraoptic and tuberomammillary nuclei and also in neurones scattered throughout the lateral hypothalamus. α_1 staining was in comparison sparser, and was principally seen in association with fine processes in the ventromedial nucleus and with individual neurones scattered throughout the lateral hypothalamus/preoptic area.

2.2.7 Midbrain Aminergic Nuclei and Colliculi

In the substantia nigra, pars reticulata, very heavy α_1-like staining was apparent on neurones and processes (Fig. 7a), presumably those of the GABAergic nigrothalamic and/or nigrotectal projections, and was seen in particularly high density in the lateral quarters of the interpeduncular nucleus, where it overlapped with the input to this nucleus of the substance P-containing projection from habenula (Fig. 7c, own observations). In contrast, the striatally projecting dopaminergic neurones of the pars compacta were very lightly stained by α_3 antiserum, like neurones of other midbrain monoaminergic nuclei such as the serotonergic dorsal and median raphe and the noradrenergic locus coeruleus (own observations and Gao et al. 1992). The midbrain also contains the location of the heaviest α_5 staining in the CNS, which was localised to the cell bodies of the primary afferent neurones of the mesencephalic trigeminal nucleus (Fig. 7b).

Complementary distributions of subunit-LIR were seen in the colliculi where α_1-LIR decorated cell bodies and presumptive dendritic processes throughout the inferior colliculus, whereas α_2 was the most prominent subunit in the superior colliculus, concentrated especially in a homogeneous staining of the most superficial layers.

2.2.8 Cerebellum

In the cerebellum, the principal immunoreactivities detected were those of α_1, seen on granule cell somata, Purkinje cell somata and on basket and stellate neurones throughout the molecular layer (Fig. 8a), and of α_6, which was confined to the cell bodies of granule cells (Fig. 8b). These distributions match those of the respective mRNAs (Laurie et al. 1992).

2.2.9 Spinal Cord

In sections of cervical and thoracic spinal cord, α_2 and α_3 were the most abundant species and were associated with motor neuronal somata in the

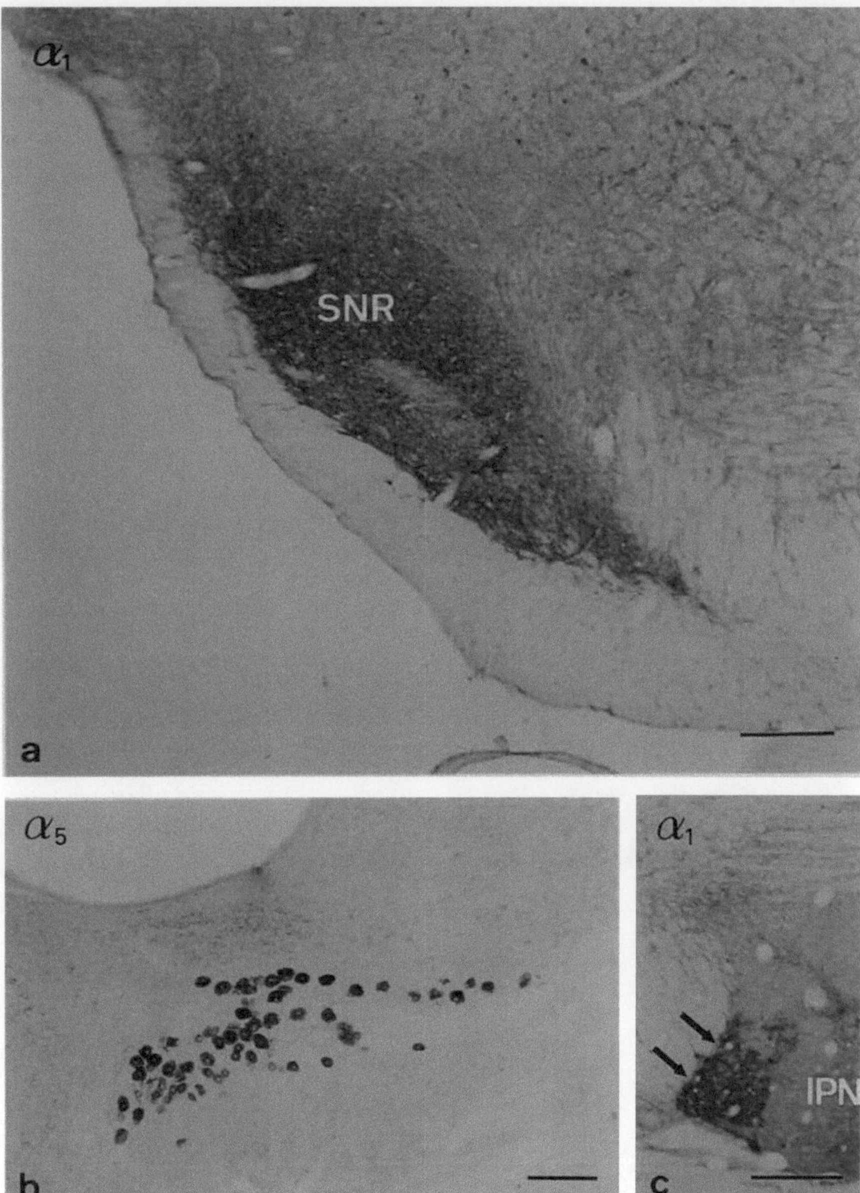

Fig. 7a–c. Midbrain. **a** The major species in the midbrain is α_1, which is present in substantia nigra, pars reticulata (*SNR*), red nucleus and cell groups throughout the mesencephalon. **b** Very intense staining with α_5 antiserum is seen in the cell bodies of primary afferent neurones in the mesencephalic trigeminal nucleus. **c** Particularly intense is the α_1 staining of the lateral aspect of the interpeduncular nucleus (*arrows*). *Scale bars* represent 500 µm (**a,c**) and 100 µm (**b**)

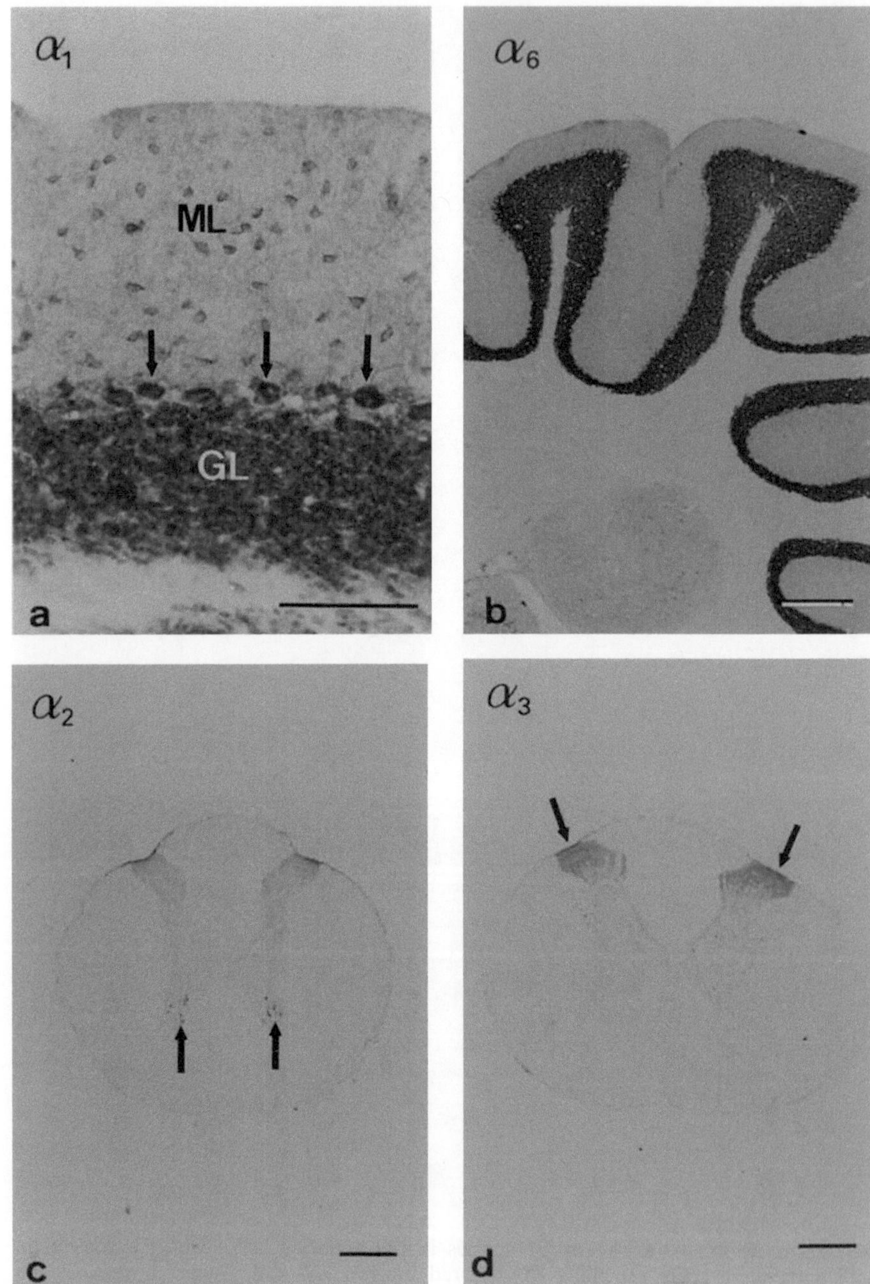

Fig. 8a–d. Cerebellum and spinal cord. **a** α_1-LIR is seen in somata in granular layer (*GL*), in Purkinje cells (*arrows*) and in basket and stellate neurones in the molecular layer (*ML*). **b** The α_6 antiserum stains cerebellar granule cell somata very intensely. **c** In the thoracic spinal cord, the major species are α_2, decorating motor neurones (*arrows*) and **d** α_3, which exhibits fine staining in the dorsal horn (*arrows*). *Scale bars* represent 200 μm (**a**) and 500 μm (**b–d**)

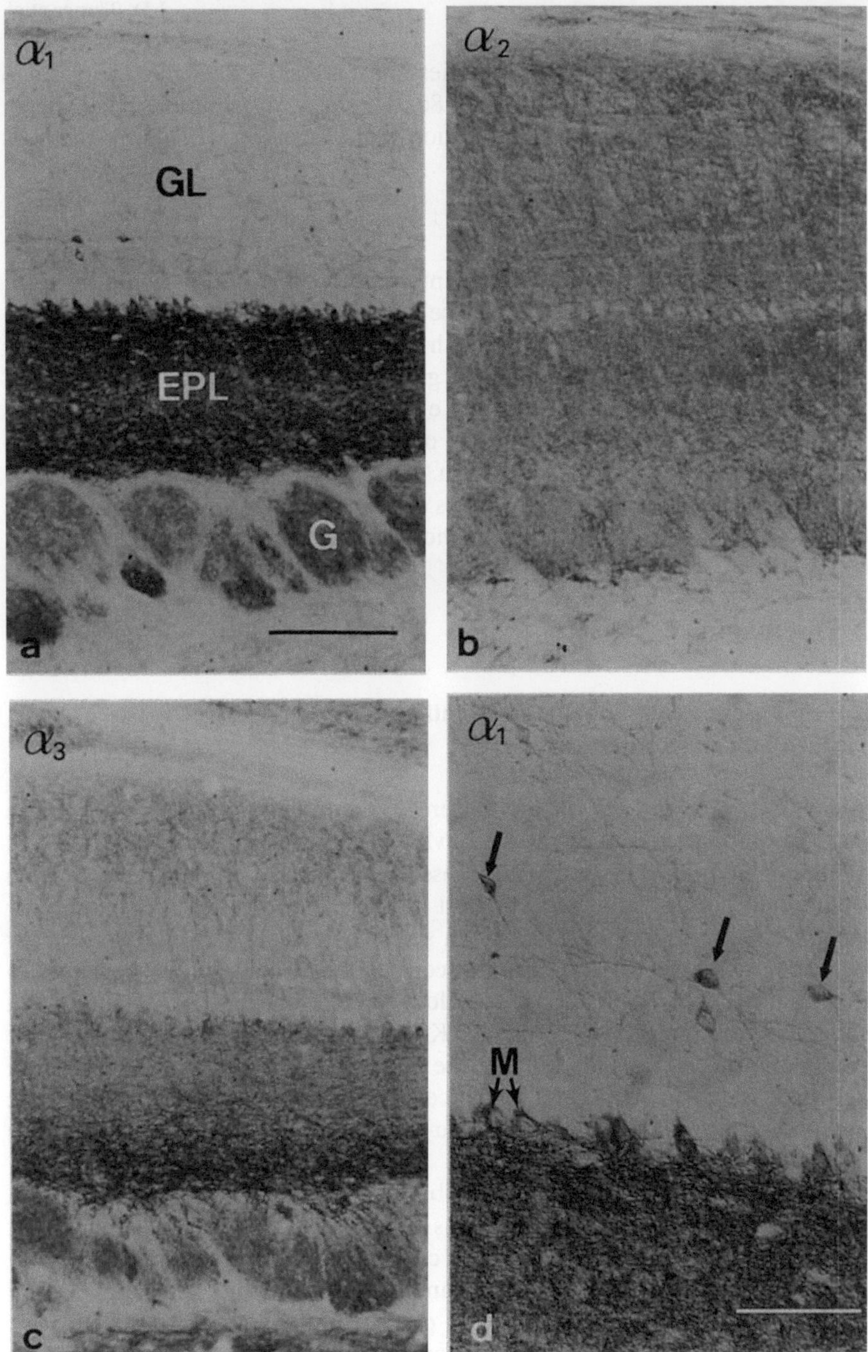

Fig. 9a–d. Olfactory bulb. **a,d** α_1-LIR is the most abundant species, associated with mitral cell somata (*M*), with processes in the external plexiform layer (*EPL*), with interneurones in the granular layer (*GL* and *arrows*) and to a lesser extent with the glomeruli (*G*). **b** In contrast, α_2-LIR is diffuse and homogeneous and the mitral cells seem unstained. **c** The distribution of α_3-LIR overlaps with that of α_1, but is less intense in the mitral cells and in the internal half of *EPL*. *Scale bars* represent 200 µm (**a–c**) and 100 µm (**d**)

ventral horn and with small cell bodies and axonal or dendritic elements in the dorsal horn, respectively (Fig. 8c,d). These distributions also match those predicted by in situ hybridisation demonstration of subunit mRNAs (Persohn et al. 1991).

2.2.10 Olfactory Bulb

In the olfactory bulb clear complementary patterns of α-LIR could be seen, although there was evidence for close colocalisation of two α subunits. α_1-LIR were prominently associated with mitral cell bodies and their dendritic trees and with interneurones in the granule cell layer (Fig. 9a,d). The α_3 antibody also stained these former elements lightly, but in addition was more concentrated on the processes of presumptive tufted cells in the external half of the external plexiform layer (Fig. 9c). In contrast to these distributions, α_2 labelled the processes of granule cells (Fig. 9b). All of these distributions can be predicted from those of the respective mRNAs.

3 Discussion

3.1 Comparison of α-Subunit Distributions: Most Receptors Contain a Single α-Subunit Species

While the distributions of the different subunits as evidenced by these antisera quite clearly overlap, the obvious differences in distribution and in quality of staining (i.e., somata/processes/particulate staining), evident even at the light microscopic level, suggest that the majority of GABA-receptor complexes in rat CNS contain only a single α species. This is supported by biochemical studies of solubilised receptors which have only been able to demonstrate the presence of a very low level of coexistence of different α subunits within receptors (e.g., McKernan et al. 1991). However, some possible locations for such coexistence have been visualised in this study, in neuronal systems such as the mitral cells of the olfactory bulb (α_1, α_3), the pyramidal cells of the hippocampus (α_2, α_5 and α_1, α_3) and the granule cells of the cerebellum (α_1, α_6).

Comparison of the global distributions of the different α-LIRs with the autoradiographic binding patterns of a variety of ligands for the BZR indicates that α_1-containing receptors codistribute with receptors of the BZ1 type, which are the most ubiquitous and have high affinity for zolpidem and β-carbolines. The sum of α_2, α_3 and α_5 distributions overlaps with that of receptors of the BZ2 type, which are less ubiquitous, with the highest relative concentrations in spinal cord, hippocampus, striatum and neocortex, and which exhibit five- to tenfold lower affinity for zolpidem and the β-carbolines (see e.g., Doble and Martin 1992; Sieghart and Schlerka 1992). Of the BZ2-type receptors, the majority are likely to contain α_2 or α_3

because α_5-LIR distribution overlaps chiefly with areas of relatively low density of BZ binding, even in hippocampus (own observations and Niddam et al. 1987; Olsen et al. 1990), and because α_5 antibodies immunoprecipitate only very small amounts of BZ binding sites in comparison with α_{1-3} antibodies (e.g., McKernan et al. 1991). The localisation of α_6-LIR exclusively to cerebellar granule cells codistributes with the unique localisation to these cells of diazepam-insensitive binding sites labelled by the imidazodiazepine Ro 15-4513 (Sieghart et al. 1987), but for which compounds from several chemical classes, including some β-carbolines, also have very high affinity (e.g., Wong and Skolnick 1992). This pharmacology is shared by recombinant receptors containing α_6 subunits (Lüddens et al. 1990), but until now the function of these sites remains obscure.

The distributions of these receptor subtypes in human brain, visualised by autoradiography using radiolabelled BZ or zolpidem as ligands, parallel those in the rat, although there are some differences, principally in the density of binding sites in some structures (e.g., Dennis et al. 1988; Hillmann and Turner, in preparation; Young and Penney 1991 and Zezula et al. 1988). For example, in cortex, high BZR densities are seen, particularly in the middle layers, and the distributions in hippocampus and densities in striatum in human and rat brain are very similar. The principal differences are in olfactory bulb, globus pallidus, substantia nigra, colliculi and septal nuclei which contain higher BZR densities in rat than in man, and in cerebellum, where, unlike in the rat, conventional BZR are at least as abundant in the granule layer as in the molecular layer in human brain.

3.2 Localisation of Different Subunits to Specific Cellular Locations or to Discrete Neuronal Systems

It is known from electrophysiological and biochemical studies (e.g., Sigel et al. 1990; Pritchett et al. 1989) that the presence of different α subunits in recombinant receptors confers different biophysical (e.g., maximal GABA-elicited conductance, desensitisation characteristics) and/or pharmacological properties (e.g., affinities of ligands for different sites on the complex).

One reason for a multiplicity of GABA-receptor subtypes could be a requirement for receptors with different biophysical properties, which permit the appropriate inhibitory effects at different locations on postsynaptic membranes (e.g., on soma, proximal dendrite, distal dendrite, spine or axon), in keeping with the highly anatomically organised GABAergic inputs onto many neuronal types (see e.g., Jones 1975; Farinas and deFelipe 1991a,b). For example, it could be speculated that the properties of a GABA receptor located on the initial axonal segment of a cortical pyramidal cell (the target of the chandelier-type interneurone) may, or may have to be different from those of a receptor located on its soma (the main target of the basket interneurone) or of a receptor located on the distal apical dendrite (target of some local circuit interneurones; for details of circuitry see White 1989). The laminar distributions of the three major cortical α subunits could fit such a scheme if α_1 locates to cell bodies and proximal dendrites especially in intermediate layers, α_2 to distal dendritic arbourisations in the superficial layers and α_3 to axonal processes in the deep layers. Perhaps clearer evidence for a cellular compartmentalisation of receptor subtypes comes from the dentate gyrus of the hippocampus where α_1 is associated with dendritic fields, α_2 to granule cell somata and dendritic fields and α_3 principally to the proximal third of the molecular layer (Fig. 3a–c) and in the Purkinje cells of cerebellum, where α_1-LIR is associated with the cell somata while α_3-LIR has been reported on somata and dendritic trees (Fritschy et al. 1992). Further studies at the electron microscope level are clearly required to identify the cellular elements labelled in these different brain areas by the different antisera.

A second reason for the existence of distinct receptor subtypes could be a requirement for receptors with different characteristics for the control of postsynaptic neurones with different intrinsic properties or with different synaptic inputs (e.g., receiving tonic GABAergic innervation, tonically active, burst firing). In this respect it is clearly demonstrable that certain neuronal groups express receptors containing a particular α species (e.g., the α_1-positive GABAergic projection neurones of the basal forebrain and substantia nigra, the α_2-positive alpha motor neurones of the spinal cord, the α_3-positive neurones of the midbrain aminergic nuclei and the α_5-positive primary afferent neurones of the mesencephalic trigeminal nucleus). This may also pertain in the neocortex where the laminar patterns of immunoreactivity could reflect localisation of particular receptor subtypes to different populations of principal or interneurones.

In summary therefore, there is evidence that individual neurones can synthesise multiple receptor subtypes and segregate them in discrete cellular locations, and also that in frequent cases specific neurone types, possibly dependent on their function, synthesise specific receptor subtypes.

3.3 Are Receptor Subtypes Responsible for Different Components of the BZ Profile?

As far as is known, the BZ as a substance class interact nonselectively with recombinant receptor subtypes (with the exception of those containing α_4 or α_6 subunits) and also with native receptor subtypes (with the exception of cerebellar diazepam-insensitive sites). An aim of defining the global distributions of the α subunit-LIRs and their association with identified neuronal systems is to attempt to relate different receptor subtypes to different features of the BZ profile (e.g., sedative, anxiolytic, anticonvulsant, amnestic, muscle relaxant or ataxic effects). Autoradiographic studies using ligands capable of distinguishing between the major BZ1 and BZ2 subtypes of BZR have shown that in the rat as well as in man, BZ1 receptors are enriched in sensorimotor brain areas, while BZ2 receptors are more densely distributed in limbic areas, although with the possible exception of the cerebellar molecular layer (BZ1) and the spinal cord (BZ2), receptor populations throughout the brain are mixed (e.g., Dennis et al. 1988; Niddam et al. 1987; Zezula et al. 1988). Thus it has been postulated that BZ1-receptor activation may be more associated with the sedative/hypnotic properties of BZ agonists, while BZ2 receptors mediate the anxiolytic/ anticonvulsant effects. The current immunocytochemical studies support this notion at least in part (e.g., the location of high density α_1-LIR to motor-related brain areas such as pallidum, substantia nigra reticulata and cerebellum, and of high concentrations of α_2 and α_3 staining in limbic areas such as amygdala, ventral striatum and hippocampus). However, it has not been possible unequivocally to associate identified receptor subtypes with different features of BZ pharmacology, principally because the distributions of the different α subunits overlap, and because the neural substrates of the respective features of the BZ activity spectrum are not yet known in sufficient detail. This may in any case be too simplistic a notion, particularly in view of the complex interactions of at least some of the neuronal systems so far identified by their likely receptor complement. An illustration of this complexity comes from the septo-hippocampal projection, where GABAergic neurones in medial septum bear α_1-containing receptors as very probably also do their target neurones in hippocampus, which themselves are GABAergic (see Freund and Antal 1988). The consequences of BZR activation for the activity of inhibitory systems arranged like these in series, and for the structures they control, are difficult to predict.

It is possible, however, to make some speculations regarding some features of the profiles of atypical compounds like abecarnil, which is markedly less muscle relaxant than BZ agonists like diazepam. Abecarnil, like other β-carbolines, shows a five- to tenfold higher affinity for receptors of the BZ1 type determined in brain membranes, but shows additional selectivity in exhibiting differing intrinsic efficacies at different recombinant receptors (see Pribilla et al., this volume). In particular, abecarnil shows high efficacy at α_3-containing receptors, which are distributed in spinal cord in the dorsal horn, but shows low efficacy at α_2-containing receptors which in spinal cord are concentrated on alpha motor neurones. This particular combination of actions at different BZ2-type receptors in spinal cord may account for the lack of efficacy of abecarnil compared with conventional BZ agonists in influencing spinal reflexes and motor coordination, and in eliciting muscle relaxation, features which should confer on the compound a pronounced advantage in the clinic.

4 Conclusion

The mapping of α subunits in the rat CNS using subunit-specific antibodies reveals distinct but overlapping distributions, which with few exceptions parallel those of their respective mRNAs, and are consistent with the presence of only a single α species in most receptors. Their distributions also match well those of the known BZR subtypes in rat brain (BZ1, BZ2 and diazepam-insensitive binding). These studies have permitted the identification of some neuronal systems which express specific receptor types and which may offer preparations for the electrophysiological and biochemical analysis of native receptors, and which may help explain some of the unusual pharmacological features of abecarnil. However, they have not permitted the clear allocation of features of the BZ agonist pharmacological profile to activation of defined receptor subtypes, but have rather reinforced the notion that for the most part this is unlikely to be the case. It is to be hoped therefore that the screening of compounds using recombinant receptors may lead in the future to the identification of more selective receptor ligands than those currently available, and that these new tools will lead to the unravelling of the functions of different GABA/BZR in the CNS.

References

Dennis T, Dubois A, Benavides J, Scatton B (1988) Distribution of central ω_1 (benzodiazepine1)- and ω_2 (benzodiazepine2)-receptor subtypes in the monkey and human brain. An autoradiographic study with [^{3}H] flunitrazepam and the ω_1-selective ligand [^{3}H] zolpidem. J Pharmacol Exp Ther 247:309–322

Doble A, Martin IL (1992) Multiple benzodiazepine receptors: no reason for anxiety. TIPS 13:76–81

Duggan MJ, Stephenson FA (1990) Biochemical evidence for the existence of γ-aminobutyrate$_A$ receptor iso-oligomers. J Biol Chem 265:3831–3835

Farinas I, deFelipe J (1991a) Patterns of synaptic input on corticocortical and corticothalamic cells in the cat visual cortex. I. The cell body. J Comp Neurol 30:53–69

Farinas I, deFelipe J (1991b) Patterns of synaptic input on corticocortical and corticothalamic cells in the cat visual cortex. II. The axon initial segment. J Comp Neurol 30:70–77

Freund T, Antal M (1988) GABA-containing neurons in the septum control inhibitory interneurons in the hippocampus. Nature 336:170–173

Fritschy JM, Benke D, Mertens S, Oertel W, Bachi T, Möhler H (1992) Five subtypes of type A γ-aminobutyric acid receptors identified in neurons by double and triple immunofluorescence staining with subunit-specific antibodies. PNAS 89:6726–6730

Gao B, Hornung JP, Fritschy JM (1992) Specific expression of the GABA$_A$-receptor α_3- but not α_1-subunit on monoaminergic and cholinergic neurons. Soc Neurosci Abstr 18:261

Gray JA (1982) The neuropsychology of anxiety. Clarendon, Oxford

Jones EG (1975) Varieties and distribution of non-pyramidal cells in the somatic sensory cortex of the squirrel monkey. J Comp Neurol 160:205–268

Kiss J, Patel AJ, Freund T (1990) Distribution of septohippocampal neurons containing parvalbumin or choline acetyl transferase in the rat brain. J Comp Neurol 298: 362–372

Laurie DJ, Seeburg PH, Wisden W (1992) The distribution of 13 GABA$_A$-receptor-subunit mRNAs in the rat brain. II. Olfactory bulb and cerebellum. J Neurosci 12:1063–1076

Lüddens H, Wisden W (1991) Function and pharmacology of multiple GABA$_A$-receptor subunits. TIPS 12:49–51

Lüddens H, Pritchett DB, Kohler M, Killisch I, Keinanen K, Monyer H, Sprengel R, Seeburg PH (1990) Cerebellar GABA$_A$-receptor selective for a behavioural alcohol antagonist. Nature 346:648–651

McKernan R, Quirk K, Prince R, Cox PA, Gillard NP, Ragan CI, Whiting P (1991) GABA$_A$-receptor subtypes immunopurified from rat brain with α-subunit antibodies have unique pharmacological properties. Neuron 7:667–676

Niddam R, Dubois A, Scatton B, Arbilla S, Langer SZ (1987) Autoradiographic localisation of [^{3}H]-zolpidem binding sites in the rat CNS: comparison with the distribution of [^{3}H]-flunitrazepam binding sites. J Neurochem 49:890–899

Olsen RW, Tobin AJ (1990) Molecular biology of GABA$_A$ receptors. FASEB J 4:1469–1480

Olsen RW, McCabe RT, Walmsley JK (1990) GABA$_A$-receptor subtypes: autoradiographic comparison of GABA, benzodiazepine and convulsant binding sites in the rat central nervous system. J Chem Neuroanat 3:59–76

Persohn E, Malherbe P, Richards JG (1991) In situ hybridisation histochemistry reveals a diversity of GABA$_A$-receptor-subunit mRNAs in neurons of the rat spinal cord and dorsal root ganglia. Neuroscience 42:497–507

Pritchett DB, Seeburg PH (1990) γ-aminobutyric acid$_A$-receptor α$_5$ subunit creates novel type II benzodiazepine receptor pharmacology. J Neurochem 54:1802–1804

Pritchett DB, Lüddens H, Seeburg PH (1989) Type I and type II GABA$_A$ receptors produced in transfected cells. Science 245:1389–1391

Sieghart W, Schlerka W (1991) Potency of several type I-benzodiazepine-receptor ligands for inhibition of [^{3}H]flunitrazepam binding in different rat brain tissues. Eur J Pharmacol 197:103–107

Sieghardt W, Eichinger A, Richards JG, Möhler H (1987) Photoaffinity labelling of Benzodiazepine receptor proteins with the partial inverse agonist [^{3}H] Ro 15-4513: a biochemical and autoradiographic study. J Neurochem 48:46–52

Sigel E, Baur R, Trube G, Möhler H, Malherbe P (1990) The effect of subunit composition of rat brain GABA$_A$ receptors on channel function. Neuron 5:703–711

Stephenson FA (1991) The GABA$_A$ receptors: structure and function. Curr Asp Neurosci 3:177–194

Thompson CL, Bodewitz G, Stephenson FA, Turner JD (1992) Mapping of GABA$_A$ receptor α$_5$- and α$_6$-subunit-like immunoreactivity in rat brain. Neurosci Lett (in press)

White EL (1989) Cortical circuits: synaptic organisation of the cerebral cortex. Structure, function and theory. Birkhauser, Boston

Wisden W, Laurie DJ, Monyer H, Seeburg PH (1992) The distribution of 13 GABA$_A$-receptor-subunit mRNAs in the rat brain. I. Telencephalon, Diencephalon, Mesencephalon. J Neurosci 12:1040–1062

Wong G, Skolnick P (1992) High-affinity ligands for "diazepam-insensitive" benzodiazepine receptors. Eur J Pharmacol 225:63–68

Young AB, Penney JB (1991) Benzodiazepine, GABA and glutamate receptors in cerebral cortex, hippocampus, basal ganglia and cerebellum. In: Mendelsohn FAO, Paxinos G (eds) Receptors in the human nervous system. Academic, New York

Zezula J, Cortes R, Probst A, Palacios JM (1988) Benzodiazepine-receptor sites in the human brain: autoradiographic mapping. Neurosci 25:771–795

Abecarnil is a Full Agonist at Some, and a Partial Agonist at Other Recombinant GABA$_A$ Receptor Subtypes

I. Pribilla[1], R. Neuhaus, R. Huba, M. Hillmann, J.D. Turner, D.N. Stephens, and H.H. Schneider

1 Introduction

γ-Aminobutyric acid (GABA) and glycine are the major inhibitory neurotransmitters in the central nervous system. Chloride influx through GABA- or glycine-gated ion channels reduces neuronal excitability. These anion channels belong to a ligand-gated ion channel family and are formed by pentamers of five membrane-spanning subunits. For the vertebrate GABA$_A$ receptor, 16 such receptor subunits, divided by sequence and functional homology into five classes called α, β, γ, δ and ρ, have been cloned. Each class consists of several subunit isotypes (for example $\alpha_1-\alpha_6$), which may differ only in few amino acids but which differ markedly in their expression patterns in the CNS, both in adulthood and during development.

Determination of the subunit composition within the pentamers representing GABA$_A$ receptors in the CNS is currently the subject of several immunoprecipitation and -purification studies. At least for the α isotypes it seems, at present, most likely that only one isotype is present in a given receptor (Duggan and Stephenson 1990; McKernan et al. 1991). From expression studies in heterologous systems (293 cells and Xenopus oocytes; see below), it is known that combinations of α and β subunits alone are sufficient to form GABA-gated chloride channels and that the addition of a γ subunit confers benzodiazepine sensitivity to the receptor complex. The pharmacological properties of the benzodiazepine site depend on the particular α and γ isotypes present in the receptor pentamer. These discoveries provide a molecular basis for the known heterogeneity of GABA$_A$ receptor pharmacology in the CNS.

2 Modulators of the GABA$_A$ Receptor

The GABA response at GABA$_A$ receptors can be modulated by several substance classes, including benzodiazepines and β-carbolines, which influence the GABA effect noncompetitively by an allosteric mechanism.

---

[1] Research Laboratories of Schering AG, 13342 Berlin, Germany

Although the exact nature of the influence is not known, the most likely explanation is that their modulation of GABA response may be achieved by altering GABA binding kinetics. Alternatively, the GABA-induced conformational change of the receptor that determines the opening of the chloride channel may be altered, thus leading to changes in conductivity or channel opening time.

Some modulators increase the receptors' response to GABA and are defined as agonistic ligands, while others decrease the GABA response and are therefore defined as inverse agonistic modulators. The substances also differ in their modulatory efficacy: "full" modulators induce strong alterations in the response to a given GABA concentration, while others induce only weak changes and are therefore called "partial" agonists or "partial" inverse agonists. Whether this modulatory efficacy is an intrinsic property of each ligand, or whether one substance may be a partial agonist at one receptor type and a full agonist at another, is still a matter of debate.

A correlation has been found, between the modulatory efficacy of a substance and the effect that GABA has on the binding affinity of this modulator: the affinity of a full modulator is strongly influenced by the presence of GABA, while the affinities of partial modulators are only weakly modified by GABA. Thus the GABA-induced shift in binding affinity of a given substance can be used as an indication of its modulatory efficacy. Furthermore, the quality of modulation is reflected by the affinity shift: agonistic modulators show increased affinities in the presence of GABA, while the affinities of inverse agonists are decreased by GABA. The affinity of a benzodiazepine such as diazepam may be increased as much as fivefold in the presence of GABA; thus the GABA ratio, defined as the ratio from the IC_{50} values determined in the absence and presence of GABA for a full agonistic modulator like diazepam, is about 5. Inverse agonists, on the other hand, like the β-carboline DMCM show GABA ratios of less than 0.5. Partial agonists and partial inverse agonists elicit intermediate GABA ratios. Substances that bind to this modulatory site on the receptor but do not influence the GABA response, the so-called benzodiazepine receptor antagonists (as they compete with other modulators for this binding site without inducing any modulation by themselves), are not influenced by GABA and therefore exhibit GABA ratios of 1.

In addition to benzodiazepine modulation of GABAergic transmission, barbiturates and some neurosteroids increase GABA-induced chloride currents via other modulatory sites on the $GABA_A$ receptor. In contrast to the benzodiazepines and β-carbolines, however, at high concentrations they act directly as agonists that induce channel openings, even in the absence of GABA. Such uncontrolled openings of the chloride channels may lead to a general breakdown of neuronal activity, including that controlling vital functions. For this reason, barbiturates have been almost entirely substituted by the benzodiazepines as hypnotics and anxiolytics.

3 GABA$_A$ Receptor Subtypes

In order to study the physiology and pharmacology of specific combinations of receptor subunits leading to subtypes of the receptor, Pritchett et al. (1988) have introduced an expression system using transformed human embryonic kidney cells (293 cells) for the production of recombinant GABA$_A$ receptors (Fig. 1): cDNAs coding for particular receptor subunits are cloned into vectors containing a strong viral promotor that allows effective transcription of the cDNA once the construct has entered a living eucaryotic cell. Vectors containing the subunit cDNAs of interest are mixed and precipitated on the 293 cells that under normal conditions do not express any GABA$_A$ receptors of their own. The precipitate covers the cells and is taken up by endocytosis. Within 48 h the cDNAs are transcribed into mRNAs that are translated into the respective polypeptides, which assemble into functional receptor complexes in the plasma membrane of the cells. These membranes containing a specific receptor type of known subunit content can then be used for binding assays.

Using this approach, it could be demonstrated that the familiar benzodiazepines differentiate between two populations of GABA$_A$ receptors: for those receptor combinations containing α_4 or α_6 subunits, benzodiazepines have low affinity, while benzodiazepines bind with similar high affinity to

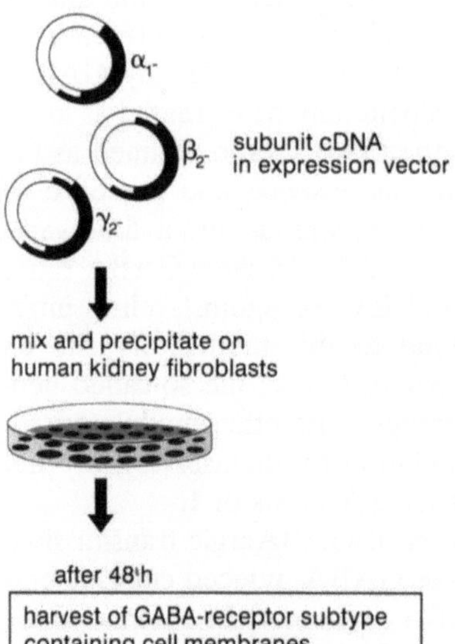

Fig. 1. GABA receptor expression in mammalian cell culture: transformed human embryonic kidney cells are transfected with GABA$_A$ receptor subunit cDNA combinations according to the CaPO$_4$ precipitation method described by Chen and Okayama (1987). Within 48 h, the polypeptides are synthesised and assembled into functional GABA$_A$ receptors in the membrane of the cells

combinations containing α_1, α_2, α_3 or α_5 isotypes (Pritchett et al. 1989; Pritchett and Seeburg 1990; Lüddens et al. 1990; Wisden et al. 1991). Nevertheless, this latter subgroup can be further differentiated: a combination of α_1, β_x and γ_2 subunits exhibits the pharmacological profile defined as the BZ I type of GABA$_A$ receptor. They are characterised by a greater affinity to the triazolopyridine CL 218 872 and the imidazopyridine zolpidem and constitute the predominant class of GABA$_A$ receptors in the CNS. BZ I receptors are present throughout the brain, while being rare in spinal cord. In contrast, BZ II receptors, which bind CL 218 872 and zolpidem with somewhat lower affinity, are well-represented in spinal cord, but absent in the cerebellum (see Turner et al., this volume). These two tissues have thus been widely used for the characterisation of BZ I and BZ II receptors.

The BZ II type binding site for CL 218 872 in brain can be mimicked by combinations of α_2, α_3 or α_5 with β_x and γ_2. However zolpidem differentiates further: while its affinities to α_2- or α_3-containing recombinant receptors fit to the data from spinal cord receptors, zolpidem's affinity to α_5-containing subunit combinations is very low (Pritchett and Seeburg 1990). Indeed, a small population of zolpidem-resistant benzodiazepine binding sites with distribution matching the expression pattern of α_5 exists in rat CNS (H. Lüddens, personal communication).

In addition to distinct BZ I and BZ II receptors, there is a diazepam-insensitive benzodiazepine binding site in the cerebellum that shows high affinity binding for the imidazobenzodiazepine Ro 15-4513. Its pharmacology is mimicked by a recombinant receptor expressed from $\alpha_6\beta_2\gamma_2$ cDNAs and its localisation matches with the expression pattern of the α_6 subunit (Lüddens et al. 1990). From these and other studies it became clear that there are more than two GABA$_A$ receptor subtypes in the brain and that the recombinant expression technique provides a powerful tool for the construction of these receptor subtypes (see also Lüddens, this volume).

4 Abecarnil at Recombinant Receptors: Subtype-Specific Binding

The β-carboline abecarnil displays a GABA shift of 1.3 at rat cortex benzodiazepine receptors, suggesting that it possesses a partial agonistic character. In animal pharmacology, abecarnil has revealed a selective action in that the compound is active in several tests predictive of anxiolytic and anticonvulsant activity, while in tests of motor coordination, in contrast to the benzodiazepine diazepam, abecarnil showed no or only weak activity (see Stephens et al., this volume). While some of these properties can be explained by partial agonism, differences in the pharmacological profile between abecarnil and certain nonselective benzodiazepine receptor partial agonists (e.g., bretazenil) suggest that abecarnil's activity at the receptor

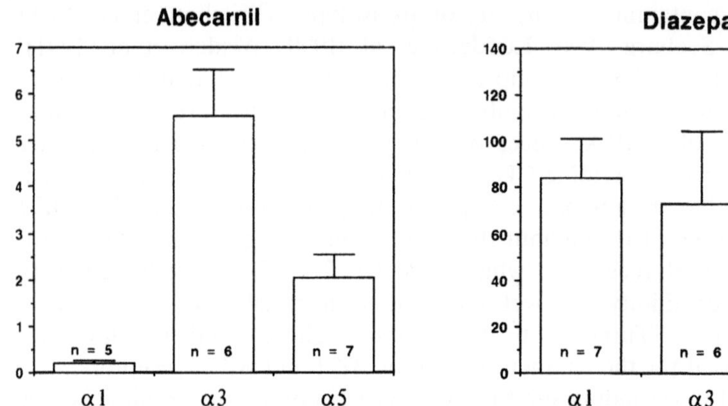

Fig. 2. Affinities of different $GABA_A$ receptor subtypes: membranes from cells transfected with either α_1 or α_3 or α_5 subunit cDNAs in combination with β_2 and γ_2 cDNAs were harvested 48 h post transfection and submitted to ^{3}H-flumazenil competition assays with abecarnil (*left*) or diazepam (*right*) as the competing drug. IC_{50} values were determined by nonlinear least square fit of the binding data. Each bar represents the mean ($\pm$ SEM) of the indicated number (*n*) of independent transfections. Specific ^{3}H-flumazenil binding was 0.2–0.6 pmol/mg membrane protein with K_D values of 5.6, 13.5 and 3.4 nM for α_1-, α_3- and α_5-containing receptors, respectively

may be more complex. To try to elucidate this, we have begun a comparison of the effects of abecarnil and diazepam at recombinant $GABA_A$ receptors expressed from different subunit–cDNA combinations. The experiments described here have focused on three pharmacologically distinct variants of recombinant receptors.

The affinities of the two drugs, abecarnil and diazepam, as determined by their ability to displace the benzodiazepine ^{3}H-flumazenil from membranes of 293 cells expressing α_1, α_3 or α_5 ($\beta_2\gamma_2$) subunit combinations are shown in Fig. 2. Abecarnil binds with 30-fold higher affinity to the α_1-containing receptor than to the α_3-containing type and displays an intermediate affinity to the α_5-containing subunit combination. In contrast, diazepam binds with similar affinity to all three receptor types tested. Depending on the receptor subtype tested, abecarnil binds with 10- to 300-fold higher affinity than diazepam. This is in agreement with data from cortical membranes where a mixed population of BZ I and BZ II receptors is present and to which abecarnil binds with about 100-fold higher affinity than diazepam.

As summarized in Table 1, abecarnil is as selective as the prototypical BZ I ligands CI 218 872 and zolpidem, which exhibit 10- to 20-fold higher affinities to α_1-containing than to α_3-containing subunit combinations. These two ligands also show about tenfold higher binding affinities to cerebellar membranes (predominantly BZ I receptors) as compared to spinal cord membranes (mainly BZ II receptors). Abecarnil shows only a fivefold higher

Table 1. Relative binding affinities of $GABA_A$ receptor ligands at cerebellar or spinal cord membranes (A) or membranes of cells transfected with the indicated subunit cDNA combinations (B)[a]

	Diazepam	Zolpidem	Cl 218 872	Abecarnil
A				
Cerebellum	1.0[b]	1.0[c]	1.0[c]	1.0[b]
Spinal cord	1.1[b]	10.5[c]	8.9[c]	5.4[b]
B				
$\alpha_1\beta_2\gamma_2$	1.0	1.0	1.0[d]	1.0
$\alpha_3\beta_2\gamma_2$	1.0	21.0	12.0[d]	30.0
$\alpha_5\beta_2\gamma_2$	1.0	>800.0	4.0[d]	6.0

[a] Values were normalised to the cerebellar or $\alpha_1\beta_2\gamma_2$ values, respectively.
[b] Stephens et al. 1992
[c] Sieghart and Schkerla 1991
[d] Pritchett and Seeburg 1990

binding affinity at the BZ I-rich cerebellar membranes when commmpared to that of BZ II containing spinal cord membranes. Since we have not yet expressed α_2-containing subunit combinations, it remains an open question whether good binding to this subtype of BZ II receptors in spinal cord accounts for the slight difference in tissue- and recombinant receptor data for abecarnil. With the relatively good binding affinity to α_5-containing receptors, abecarnil's specificity profile resembles that of the triazolopyridine CI 218 872.

As some β-carbolines exhibit relatively good binding affinities at the diazepam-insensitive benzodiazepine binding site (DIB) in the cerebellum (Turner et al. 1991), it appeared to be possible that some of abecarnil's pharmacological effects might be mediated via this site. For this reason abecarnil's binding affinity was determined by its ability to displace ^{3}H-Ro15-4513 from the diazepam-sensitive and -insensitive sites in the cerebel-

Table 2. Relative binding affinities of $GABA_A$ receptor ligands at the diazepam-sensitive (DSB) and -insensitive (DIB) benzodiazepine binding site of cerebellar membranes or membranes of cells transfected with the indicated subunit cDNA combination[a]

	Diazepam	Abecarnil	Bretazenil
DSB	1.0	1.0	1.0
DIB	>1000.0	245.0	18.0
$\alpha_1\beta_2\gamma_2$	1.0	1.0	n.d.
$\alpha_6\beta_2\gamma_2$[b]	>200.0	1000.0	n.d.

[a] IC_{50} values were determined for displacement of ^{3}H-Ro15-4513 and were normalized to the DSB site or the $\alpha_1\beta_2\gamma_2$ combination, respectively.
[b] Data for abecarnil at α_6-containing receptors are from a personal communication from H. Wieland and P. Seeburg.

lum and from recombinant receptors assembled from α_1 or α_6 ($\beta_2\gamma_2$) subunit cDNA combinations. As shown in Table 2, abecarnil, like diazepam, binds to the DIB site and its recombinant counterpart only with very low affinity, so it is unlikely that this site is involved in abecarnil's pharmacological effects. Abecarnil differs in this respect from another partial agonist of the $GABA_A$ receptor, bretazenil, that binds with relatively high affinity at the DIB site.

5 Abecarnil at Recombinant Receptors: Are There Subtype-Specific Effects?

While differential binding affinity represents one form of selectivity for receptors, it may not be the only factor, because receptor subtype specific differences in modulatory efficacy may also be possible. To obtain information on the modulatory efficacy of abecarnil and diazepam, the competition experiments (i.e., the ability to displace ^{3}H-flumazenil) were carried out in the presence and absence of $30\,\mu M$ GABA and the shifts of the IC_{50} values were expressed as the "GABA ratios" ($IC_{50} - GABA/IC_{50} + GABA$; Fig. 3). Diazepam, predicted to be a full agonist at all $GABA_A$ receptors, showed GABA ratios significantly above 2 for all three types of recombinant receptors tested. The binding of abecarnil to the α_1- and α_5-containing combinations was weakly affected by GABA, but it displayed a more distinct GABA-induced affinity shift at receptors assembled from the $\alpha_3\beta_2\gamma_2$ subunit combination. Does that reflect different modulatory efficacies at these different receptor subtypes?

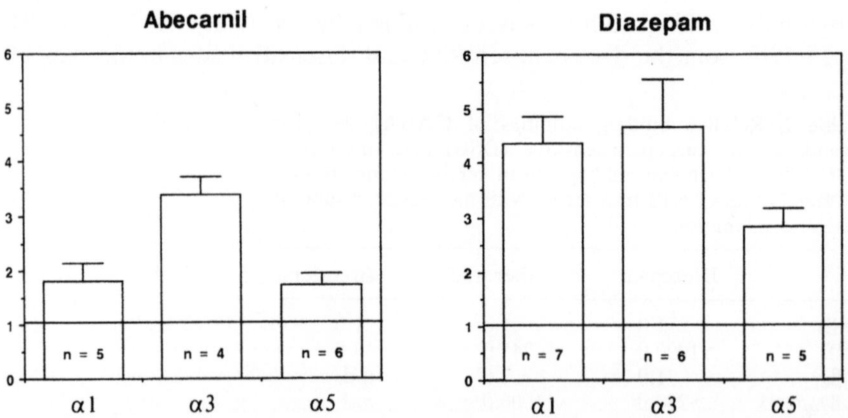

Fig. 3. GABA ratios at different $GABA_A$ receptor subtypes: the GABA-induced affinity shift for the two modulatory drugs is expressed as the ratio of IC_{50} values determined in the absence and presence of $30\,\mu M$ GABA of membranes prepared from cells transfected with α_1, α_3 or α_5 ($\beta_2\gamma_2$) subunit combinations. Each bar represents the mean ($\pm$ SEM) of the indicated number (n) of independent transfection experiments

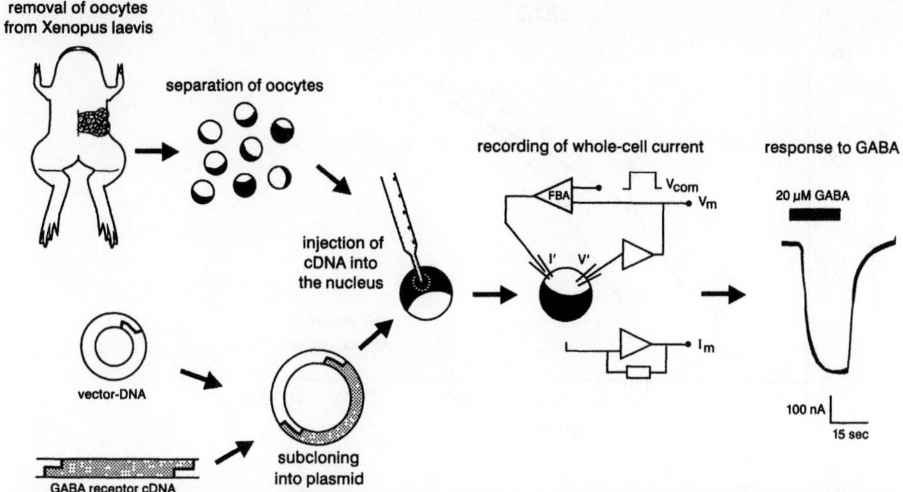

Fig. 4. GABA$_A$ receptor expression in Xenopus oocytes: oocytes are isolated from ovaries of Xenopus laevis and injected individually with different combinations of GABA$_A$ receptor α-, β- and γ-subunit cDNAs subcloned in mammalian expression vectors. 48 h after injection GABA-induced inward currents are measured in the voltage clamp mode

GABA ratios have been considered to provide a useful guide to the intrinsic efficacies of compounds acting at the benzodiazepine receptor with respect to sorting them into agonists, antagonists or inverse agonists. For distinction between partial and full agonists, however, more evidence of their ability to modulate the *function* of the receptor may be necessary to permit reliable interpretation. Functional determination of the efficacy of modulators of GABAergic signal transmission can be achieved by assessing their effects on GABA-induced chloride flux. It is possible to analyse this electrophysiologically for receptor subtypes expressed in Xenopus oocytes which have been injected with cDNAs coding for α, β and γ subunits (Fig. 4). In such cells, when their membrane potentials are clamped to $-80\,$mV, GABA induces a dose-dependent inward current.

The GABA concentration eliciting a half-maximal response was $27\,\mu M$ in Xenopus oocytes expressing the $\alpha_1\beta_2\gamma_2$ and $116\,\mu M$ in those expressing the $\alpha_3\beta_2\gamma_2$ combination. The respective GABA EC$_{10}$'s (the GABA concentration eliciting 10% of the maximal GABA response) were then applied together with increasing concentrations of abecarnil or diazepam. The resulting increase in current above the response level to GABA alone was plotted as % potentiation against the modulator concentration (Fig. 5). Diazepam potentiated the chloride flux through α_1- and α_3-containing receptors with nearly equal potencies (EC$_{50}$ diaz approximately 40 vs. $60\,$nM). In agreement with the binding data from the transfected 293 cells, abecarnil potentiated the effect of GABA at the α_1-containing receptor at lower

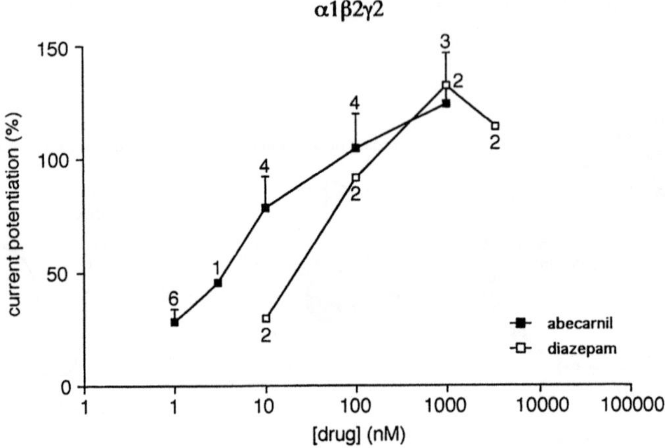

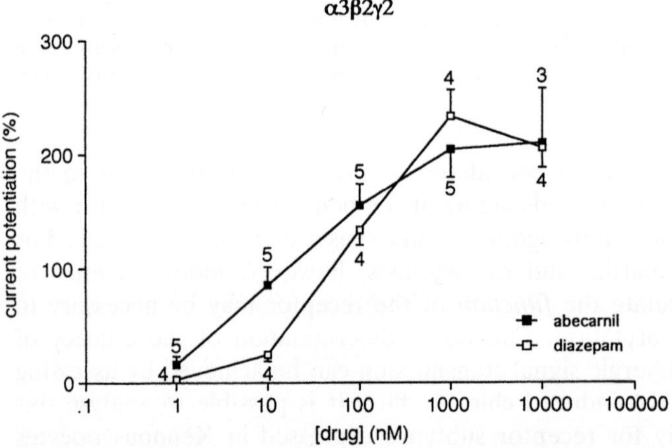

Fig. 5. Potentiation of GABA response: GABA-induced chloride currents are potentiated by increasing concentrations of the two drugs. Each point represents the mean ($\pm$ SEM) of the indicated number of independent determinations

concentrations than at the α_3-containing receptor (EC_{50} abec approximately 5 vs. 27 nM). Although the absolute EC_{50} values differ slightly from those obtained by the binding assays, these electrophysiological measurements confirmed that abecarnil is more potent than diazepam at both receptor subtypes.

The maximal potentiation achieved with abecarnil at the α_1- and the α_3-containing combination was similar to that obtained by diazepam. Thus abecarnil seems to be a full agonist at both receptor subtypes. In another electrophysiological study, abecarnil's efficacy in potentiation of GABA responses was compared to that of flunitrazepam at α_3- and $\alpha_5(\beta_2\gamma_2)$ combinations expressed in 293 cells (Knoflach et al. 1992). In this study, abecarnil showed again full agonistic activity at the α_3-containing receptor type, but was a partial agonist at the α_5-containing receptor. Finally, data from a third electrophysiological study indicate that abecarnil may also be a partial agonist at α_2-containing receptors expressed in the Xenopus system (K. Wafford, personal communication). While in the electrophysiological study using 293 cells a GABA ratio of 1.7 correlates with partial agonism (at α_5 receptors), in our investigation using the Xenopus system, a GABA ratio of 1.8 – obtained in binding studies using the 293 cell expression system – corresponds to full agonistic properties (at the α_1 receptor).

The differences in GABA ratios observed in 293 cells expressing α_1-, α_3- or α_5-containing receptors do therefore not consistently reflect the functional modification induced by abecarnil at these receptor subtypes. This can be interpreted in two ways:

1. β-carboline interaction with the $GABA_A$ receptor differs to that of benzodiazepines, so that the "GABA-ratio to modulatory efficacy-correlation" that has been established for benzodiazepines does not hold true for β-carbolines (i.e., the weak allosteric affinity rise for abecarnil induced by GABA at α_1 receptors does not correlate with a respectively weak increase in GABA affinity induced by abecarnil); or
2. the recombinant receptors produced in the Xenopus and the 293 cell system differ in their ability to be modulated (i.e., because of different posttranslational modification or different subunit stöchiometry).

Further experiments are required to test these possibilities. So far, the GABA ratio appears less useful for distinguishing partial from full agonism in recombinant receptors.

The findings that abecarnil exerts partial agonistic effects at some and full agonistic effects at other receptor subtypes stand in contrast to data with bretazenil – another partial agonist at the benzodiazepine receptor – which

Table 3. Efficacies of diazepam, abecarnil and bretazenil in modulating GABA-induced chloride flux in recombinant systems expressing subtypes of $GABA_A$ receptors in which the nature of the α-subunit was varied in combination with $\beta_x\gamma_2$

	α_1	α_2	α_3	α_5
Diazepam[a]	full	full	full	full
Abecarnil	full	partial[b]	full[c]	partial[c]
Bretazenil[a]	partial	partial	partial	partial

[a] Data for diazepam and bretazenil are from Piua et al. (1992)
[b] K. Wafford, personal communication
[c] Knoflach et al. 1992

is significantly less effective than full agonistic benzodiazepines at all subunit combinations so far tested (including α_1-, α_2-, α_3-, α_5-$\beta_x\gamma_2$ combinations; Puia et al. 1992 and Knoflach et al. 1992). Thus for some drugs partial agonism appears to be an intrinsic property of the ligand – regardless of the receptor subtype it is acting on. For abecarnil, this seems not to be the case: it rather acts receptor subtype specific with respect to both potency and modulatory efficacy.

The question remains, whether the distinct in vivo pharmacological profile of abecarnil (see Stephens et al., this volume) can be accounted for by its selectivity, in terms of differential affinity or/and of differential modulatory efficacy at particular subtypes of $GABA_A$ receptor. While this most probably is the case, it is still too early to ascribe any particular quality of abecarnil to its action at particular subtypes of receptor. The currently available data need to be completed and extended to other receptor subtypes, containing, for instance, other isoforms of β and γ subunits. Nevertheless, the complexity of possible interactions between ligands for the modulatory site of central $GABA_A$ receptors points to the possibility of finetuning of drug discovery to provide compounds with very specific pharmacological effects. Abecarnil is one of the very first of such compounds.

References

Chen C, Okayama H (1987) High-efficiency transformation of mammalian cells by plasmid DNA. Mol Cell Biol 7:2745–2751

Duggan MJ, Stephenson FA (1990) Biochemical evidence for the existence of γ-aminobutyrate$_A$ receptor iso-oligomers. J Biol Chem 265:3831–3835

Knoflach F, Drescher U, Scheurer L, Malherbe P, Möhler H (1992) Full and partial agonism displayed by benzodiazepine receptor ligands at different recombinant $GABA_A$ receptor subtypes. J Neurosci (submitted)

Lüddens H, Pritchett DB, Köhler M, Killisch I, Keinänen K, Monyer H, Sprengel R, Seeburg PH (1990) Cerebellar $GABA_A$ receptor selective for a behavioural alcohol antagonist. Nature 346:648–651

McKernan RM, Quirk K, Prince R, Cox PA, Gillard NP, Ragan CI, Whiting P (1991) $GABA_A$ receptor subtypes immunopurified from rat brain with subunit-specific antibodies have unique pharmacological properties. Neuron 7:667–676

Pritchett DB, Seeburg PH (1990) γ-aminobutyric acid A receptor α_5-subunit creates novel type II benzodiazepine receptor pharmacology. J Neurochem 54:1802–1804

Pritchett DB, Sontheimer H, Gorman CM, Kettenmann H, Seeburg PH, Scofield PR (1988) Transient expression shows ligand gating and allosteric potentiation of $GABA_A$ receptor subunits. Science 242:1306–1308

Pritchett DB, Lüddens H, Seeburg PH (1989) Type I and type II $GABA_A$-benzodiazepine receptors produced in transfected cells. Science 245:1389–1392

Puia G, Ducic I, Vicini S, Costa E (1992) Molecular mechanisms of the partial allosteric modulatory effects of bretazenil at γ-aminobutyric acid type A receptor. Proc Natl Acad Sci USA 89:3620–3624

Sieghart W, Schkerla W (1991) Potency of several type I-benzodiazepine receptor ligands for inhibition of ^{3}H-flunitrazepam binding in different rat brain tissues. Eur J Pharmacol 197:103–107

Stephens DN, Turski L, Hillman M, Turner JD, Schneider HH, Yamaguchi M (1992) What are the differences between abecarnil and conventional benzodiazepine anxiolytics? GABAergic Synaptic Transmission. Adv Biochem Psychopharmacol 47: 395–407

Turner DM, Sapp DW, Olsen RW (1991) The benzodiazepine/alcohol antagonist Ro 15-4513: binding to a $GABA_A$ receptor subtype that is insensitive to diazepam. J Pharmacol Exp Ther 257:1236–1242

Wisden W, Herb A, Wieland H, Keinänen K, Lüddens H, Seeburg PH (1991) Cloning, pharmacological characteristics and expression pattern of the rat $GABA_A$ receptor α_4 subunit. FEBS Lett 289:227–230

Pharmacological Evidence for Full Agonist Activity of Abecarnil at Certain GABA$_A$ Receptors

M. Serra, C.A. Ghiani, C. Motzo, and G. Biggio

1 Introduction

It is now well established that the degree of activation of the central γ-aminobutyric acid type A (GABA$_A$)-receptor complex is predictive of the pharmacological efficacy and clinical profile of the agonist ligands for benzodiazepine recognition sites (see review Biggio and Costa 1990; Biggio et al. 1992). Accordingly, anxiolytic and anticonvulsant drugs which enhance the function of GABAergic transmission with a low intrinsic activity are classified as "partial agonists," i.e., compounds able to reduce the risk of tolerance, dependence, and unwanted effects attributed to "full agonists."

The presence of multiple GABA$_A$ receptors in the mammalian brain (Pritchett et al. 1989a,b; Pritchett and Seeburg 1990; Luddens and Wisden 1991) has recently suggested the possibility that the activation of a subpopulation of such receptors by selective drugs might also induce a pharmacological effects more specific than those elicited by drugs which do not discriminate among the different subpopulations of receptors.

The β-carboline derivative abecarnil has recently been proposed as a new anxioselective and anticonvulsant partial agonist, with high affinity for a subpopulation of benzodiazepine recognition sites. In accordance with this pharmacological profile, this compound has been shown to induce fewer side effects (sedative effects, motor impairment, dependence etc.) than classical benzodiazepines (Stephens et al. 1990; Turski et al. 1990; Löscher et al. 1990).

Using different biochemical and pharmacological tests, we tried to clarify further the pharmacological efficacy of abecarnil at the level of the GABA$_A$-receptor complex. We mainly performed in vitro and in vivo studies using a biochemical (t-[^{35}S]butylsbicyclophosphorothioanate, [^{35}S]TBPS, binding) and pharmacological (seizure pattern) test currently used to evaluate the functional state of the central GABA$_A$–receptor complex. We also studied the action of abecarnil on GABAergic transmission in the brain of animals pretreated with isoniazid, an inhibitor of GABA

Department of Experimental Biology "Bernardo Loddo", Chair of Pharmacology, University of Cagliari, Italy synthesis (Horton et al. 1979) able to enhance [^{35}S]TBPS binding in the rat brain in a dose-related manner and to induce tonic/clonic seizures in rats and mice (Horton 1980). Thus, the animals treated with this drug represent a model to simultaneously study both the pharmacological efficacy and capability of putative anxiolytic drugs to enhance the GABAergic transmission.

2 In Vitro Studies

2.1 [^{3}H]Flunitrazepam Binding, [^{3}H]GABA Binding, and ^{36}Cl$^-$ Uptake

The finding that anxiolytic benzodiazepines exert their pharmacological effects by enhancing the interaction of GABA with its recognition site has received direct biochemical support by the finding that benzodiazepines increase [^{3}H]GABA binding and muscimol-stimulated chloride uptake in the rat brain (see for review Biggio et al. 1990). More recently, different studies have shown that most of the anxiolytic and anticonvulsant benzodiazepine recognition-site ligands, even with a chemical structure unrelated to benzodiazepines, are able to enhance both [^{3}H]GABA binding and ^{36}Cl$^-$ uptake in rat cortical membrane preparations. These data suggest that the measurement of these parameters can be used as a suitable biochemical tool to investigate, in vitro, the molecular action and efficacy of putative benzodiazepine recognition-site ligands at the level of the GABA$_A$–receptor complex.

Abecarnil displaced [^{3}H]flunitrazepam binding with a K_i of 0.46 nM, suggesting that this compound binds with high affinity to central benzodiazepine recognition sites (Fig. 1). This evidence is consistent with a previous finding by Stephens et al. (1990).

As shown in Table 1, abecarnil significantly enhanced specific [^{3}H]GABA binding in the rat cerebral cortex. The maximal increase (+35% over control) was obtained at 3 µM. In agreement with previous reports (Skerritt et al. 1982; Biggio et al. 1984), a similar enhancement can be obtained with a higher concentration (100 µM) of diazepam (Table 1). In accordance with its pharmacological characterization as a partial agonist, bretazenil (Haefely 1984) showed very weak efficacy in stimulating [^{3}H]GABA binding (+14%), even at a very high concentration (100 µM). Moreover, this compound was able to antagonize the enhancing effect of abecarnil and diazepam on [^{3}H]GABA binding (data not shown).

These results suggest that abecarnil, like diazepam, is acting as a full agonist rather than a partial agonist at the benzodiazepine recognition site in rat cortex. This conclusion is further supported by the finding that abecarnil enhanced muscimol-stimulated ^{36}Cl$^-$ uptake (Table 1) in tissue preparation from the rat cerebral cortex with an efficacy similar to diazepam and much greater than that of bretazenil. Accordingly, 10 µM abecarnil and diazepam

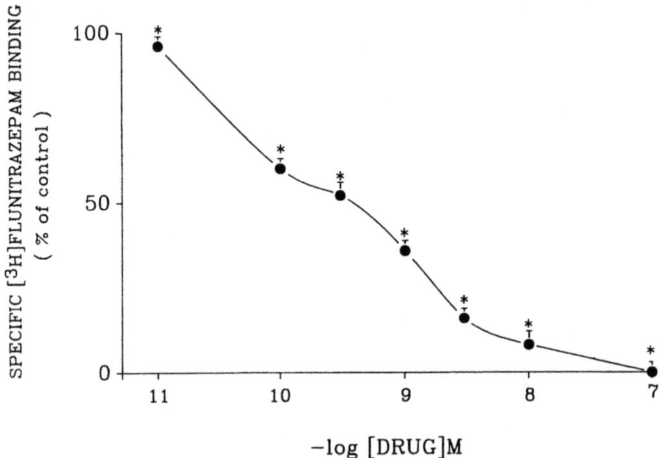

Fig. 1. Effect of abecarnil on the specific binding of [³H]flunitrazepam in the rat cerebral cortex. [³H]flunitrazepam binding to rat cortical membranes was performed as previously described (Corda et al. 1988). Each value is the mean ± standard error of mean of three separate experiments. *$p < 0.01$ compared with the control value (Student's t test)

Table 1. Effect of abecarnil, diazepam, and bretazenil on [³H]GABA binding and muscimol-stimulated ^{36}Cl⁻ uptake in the rat cerebral cortex

Drugs	(μM)	[³H]GABA binding (% of increase)	(μM)	5μM Muscimol-stimulated ^{36}Cl⁻ uptake (% of increase)
Abecarnil	3	35 ± 2.9*	10	36 ± 2.1*
Diazepam	100	39 ± 3.0*	10	39 ± 3.2*
Bretazenil	100	14 ± 1.5*	100	14 ± 2.2*

[³H]GABA binding and ^{36}Cl⁻ uptake were measured as previously described (Biggio et al. 1989). Data are expressed as percentage increase over control values. Each value is the mean ± standard error of mean of four separate experiments.
*$p < 0.01$ compared with the control value (Student's t test).

increased 5 μM muscimol-stimulated ^{36}Cl⁻ uptake by 35%–40%, while a higher concentration (100 μM) of bretazenil was only able to elicit a maximum enhancement of 14% (Table 1).

These in vitro findings showing that abecarnil increased [³H]GABA binding and muscimol-stimulated chloride uptake by an extent similar to that of diazepam strongly suggest that abecarnil can be considered a full agonist at the benzodiazepine recognition site in rat cortex.

2.2 [³⁵S]TBPS Binding in Washed and Unwashed Membranes

It is generally accepted that the cage convulsant [³⁵S]TBPS, which binds to a specific recognition site associated with the GABA-dependent chloride channel, is a useful radioligand to investigate the properties of the $GABA_A$–receptor complex. Accordingly, [^{35}S]TBPS binding is potently inhibited by drugs which facilitate the opening of the chloride channel such as benzodiazepines, GABA, and GABA mimetics, while it is affected in the opposite manner by drugs which inhibit GABAergic transmission (Squires et al. 1983; Supavilai and Karobath 1984; Gee et al. 1986; Concas et al. 1988).

The effect of benzodiazepines on [^{35}S]TBPS binding is still controversial. It has been reported that while diazepam, like GABA mimetics, decreases [^{35}S]TBPS binding in unwashed membranes (in the presence of GABA), it increases this binding in well-washed membrane preparations (devoid of GABA). On the basis of this evidence, we thought it interesting to study the effect of abecarnil on [^{35}S]TBPS binding, either in the presence or absence of GABA, comparing it to the effect of diazepam and bretazenil.

As shown in Table 2, abecarnil and diazepam decreased [^{35}S]TBPS binding with a potency and efficacy similar to diazepam and much higher than bretazenil in a concentration-dependent manner. The maximal degree of inhibition of [^{35}S]TBPS binding to unwashed rat cortical membrane preparations induced by abecarnil and diazepam was 60% and 67% at $30\,\mu M$, respectively. In contrast, consistent with its partial agonist profile, up to $30\,\mu M$ bretazenil only modified [^{35}S]TBPS binding slightly.

Together these findings further suggest that abecarnil, like diazepam, decreases [^{35}S]TBPS binding with a full agonist efficacy. This conclusion is consistent with the evidence that in some behavioral models (antagonism to

Table 2. Effect of abecarnil, diazepam, and bretazenil on [^{35}S]TBPS binding in unwashed and washed rat cortical membrane preparations

Unwashed membranes		
Drugs	Concentration (μM)	[^{35}S]TBPS binding (% of change)
Abecarnil	30	-60 ± 8*
Diazepam	30	-67 ± 7*
Bretazenil	30	-29 ± 5*

Washed membranes		
Drugs	Concentration (μM)	[^{35}S]TBPS binding (% of change)
Abecarnil	3–100	$+4 \pm 0.8$
Diazepam	3	$+35 \pm 2.0$*
Bretazenil	3–100	$+5 \pm 0.2$
Diazepam + Abecarnil	3 10	-9 ± 1.1
Diazepam + Bretazenil	3 10	-5 ± 0.9

[^{35}S]TBPS binding to unwashed and washed rat cortical membranes was performed as previously described (Concas et al. 1990). Each value is the mean $\pm$ standard error of mean of four separate experiments.

*$p < 0.01$ compared with the control value (Student's t test).

seizures induced by DMCM or audiogenic stimulation, Turski et al. 1990; anxiolytic action, Stephens et al. 1990), abecarnil is effective at fractional receptor occupancies lower than that required by diazepam (see Stephens et al., this volume).

As previously reported (Concas et al. 1990), diazepam added to membranes devoid of GABA elicited a concentration-dependent increase in [^{35}S]TBPS binding, an effect opposite to that observed using unwashed membranes (Table 2). In contrast, abecarnil and the partial agonist bretazenil failed to change significantly the binding of [^{35}S]TBPS in this membrane preparation. Moreover, both drugs completely abolished the enhancement of [^{35}S]TBPS binding elicited by diazepam. The latter effect is consistent with the concept that a partial agonist blocks the effect of a full agonist if the full agonist response measured is greater than the maximal response that can be elicited by the partial agonist alone. Thus, this evidence may suggest a partial agonist profile of abecarnil in this experimental model.

The pharmacological action of benzodiazepines is strictly dependent on the presence of GABA at the synaptic cleft. Thus, the reduced availability of GABA at the synaptic level results in a reduction or loss of the pharmacological efficacy of these drugs (Polc and Haefely 1976; Biggio et al. 1977; Gallager 1978).

On the basis of these considerations, it is tempting to speculate that the increase in [^{35}S]TBPS binding induced by diazepam in well-washed membranes (devoid of GABA) might reflect a negative or paradoxical response of this drug comparable to the paradoxical behavioral effects (increased anxiety, aggression, hostility etc.) elicited by benzodiazepines in some elderly patients, as well as in children affected by cerebral lesions (Greenblatt and Shader 1976).

In conclusion, our results indicate that abecarnil recognizes the same populations of receptors recognized by diazepam, but in contrast to the latter it fails to induce a negative effect on [^{35}S]TBPS binding. It remains to be established whether the lack of intrinsic activity of abecarnil in membranes devoid of GABA is relevant for the selective pharmacological action of this drug.

3 In Vivo Studies

3.1 [^{35}S]TBPS Binding Ex Vivo

To better clarify the intrinsic efficacy of abecarnil on the function of the GABA-coupled chloride channel, we studied whether this drug was able, like diazepam and other positive modulators of GABAergic transmission, to reduce [^{35}S]TBPS binding after in vivo administration. We have recently demonstrated that the ex vivo binding of [^{35}S]TBPS is a sensitive tool to

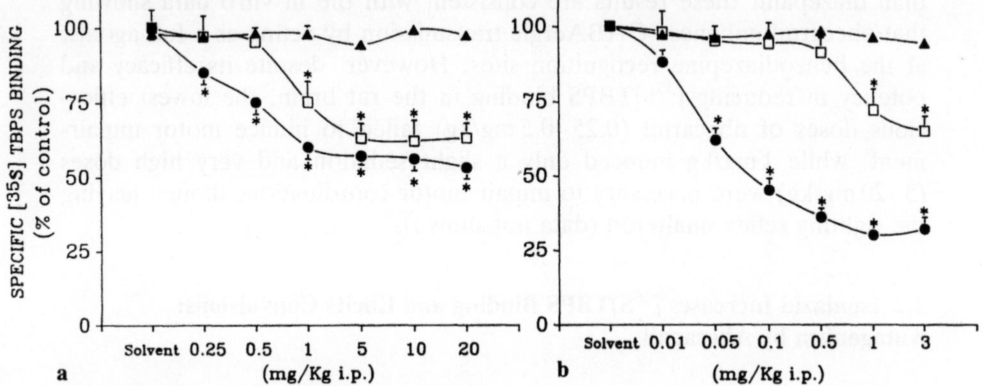

Fig. 2a–b. The i.p. administration of abecarnil induces a dose-related decrease in [^{35}S] TBPS binding in the **a** rat and **b** mouse cerebral cortex. Animals were killed 30 min after the administration of drugs or solvent. Data are expressed as percentage of solvent-treated animals. Values are the mean ± standard error of mean of five separate experiments. *$p < 0.01$ vs. solvent-treated animals (analysis of variance followed by Scheffe's test). ●, abecarnil; □, diazepam; ▲, bretazenil

identify modulators of central GABAergic synapses with different intrinsic activity in enhancing the function of GABA-coupled chloride channel (Serra et al. 1989; Biggio et al. 1990; Sanna et al. 1991). The results of this study should indicate more clearly whether abecarnil enhances GABAergic function with an efficacy similar to the full agonist diazepam, or the partial agonist bretazenil.

As shown in Fig. 2, the acute administration of abecarnil to rat or mouse induced within 30 min a dose-dependent decrease in [^{35}S]TBPS binding measured ex vivo in unwashed cortical membrane preparations. Abecarnil started to significantly decrease [^{35}S]TBPS binding in the rat cerebral cortex at the dose of 0.25 mg/kg, its effect was maximal (−40%) at the dose of 1 mg/kg, and higher doses (up to 20 mg/kg) failed to further decrease [^{35}S]TBPS binding. As previously reported (Concas et al. 1991), diazepam at the dose of 0.5 mg/kg i.p. failed to affect [^{35}S]TBPS binding in the rat cerebral cortex while its maximal effect (−25% to −30%) was obtained at the dose of 3 mg/kg i.p. In contrast, abecarnil was able to induce a comparable decrease in [^{35}S]TBPS binding at the dose of 0.5 mg/kg, six times lower than diazepam.

The abecarnil-induced decrease in [^{35}S]TBPS binding was more evident in the mouse than in the rat brain. In fact, as shown in Fig. 2, this effect was significant at a dose as low as 0.01 mg/kg i.p. and was maximal at 1 mg/kg (−70%). In contrast, bretazenil failed to reduce [^{35}S]TBPS binding in the brain of both rats and mice (Fig. 2).

Since the in vivo administration of this β-carboline enhances the function of GABA-coupled chloride channels with a potency and efficacy greater than diazepam, these results are consistent with the in vitro data showing that abecarnil enhances GABAergic transmission by acting as a full agonist at the benzodiazepine recognition sites. However, despite its efficacy and potency in reducing $[^{35}S]$TBPS binding in the rat brain, the lowest efficacious doses of abecarnil (0.25–0.5 mg/kg) failed to induce motor impairment, while 1 mg/kg induced only a slight sedation and very high doses (5–20 mg/kg) were necessary to impair motor coordination, though leaving the righting reflex unaltered (data not shown).

3.2 Isoniazid Increases $[^{35}S]$TBPS Binding and Elicits Convulsions: Antagonism by Abecarnil

Isoniazid-treated rats represent a useful model to evaluate biochemically and pharmacologically both the reduced function of the GABA-dependent chloride channel elicited by the decreased availability of GABA at the GABA recognition site, and the efficacy of anxiolytic and anticonvulsant drugs to enhance the GABAergic transmission.

Isoniazid, an inhibitor of GABA synthesis (Horton et al. 1979), produces a functional inhibition of central GABAergic transmission and this in turn elicits proconvulsant and convulsant effects and markedly increases $[^{35}S]$TBPS binding in the rat brain (Horton 1980; Serra et al. 1989). Thus, the ex vivo measurement of $[^{35}S]$TBPS binding to unwashed cortical membrane preparations and the pattern of seizures induced by isoniazid were used to study the pharmacological efficacy of abecarnil at the $GABA_A$–receptor complex.

As shown in Table 3, the subcutaneous injection of isoniazid (350 mg/kg) induced tonic/clonic seizures within 60 min and markedly enhanced $[^{35}S]$TBPS binding in the rat brain. Abecarnil (0.5 mg/kg i.p.) administered 30 min after isoniazid completely prevented the increase in $[^{35}S]$TBPS bind-

Table 3. Isoniazid induces tonic/clonic seizures and increases $[^{35}S]$TBPS binding in rat: antagonism by abecarnil

Treatment	Latency of convulsions (min)	Pattern of convulsions		$[^{35}S]$TBPS binding % of control
		Clonus	Tonus	
Isoniazid	65 ± 2	13/15[a]	7/15	147
Isoniazid + Abecarnil	77[b]	1/15*	0/15	102**

Abecarnil (0.5 mg/kg) or saline were administered i.p. 30 min after isoniazid (350 mg/kg s.c.). Pattern of convulsions (clonus/tonus) are expressed as the number of rats affected for the total number of animals in the given group.

*$p < 0.01$ vs. isoniazid-treated rats (Fisher's exact probability test); **$p < 0.01$ vs. isoniazid-treated rats (analysis of variance followed by Scheffe's test).

[a] Total number of animals in the given group.

[b] Only one rat out of 15 had convulsions 77 min after injection.

ing induced by the latter. Moreover, the same dose of abecarnil was able to antagonize the convulsions elicited by isoniazid. A similar effect was obtained with a higher dose (3 mg/kg i.p.) of diazepam, while bretazenil at a dose of 5 mg/kg i.p. did not affect $[^{35}S]TBPS$ binding and only partially antagonized the convulsions induced by isoniazid (data not shown). It is interesting to note that abecarnil antagonized both the increase in $[^{35}S]TBPS$ binding and the convulsions at a dose as low as 0.5 mg/kg, which per se failed to significantly induce any apparent motor alteration.

The capability of abecarnil to antagonize both the increase in $[^{35}S]TBPS$ binding and the seizures induced by isoniazid in rat and mice strongly suggests a good correlation between the pharmacological efficacy of the drug and its marked action in enhancing the GABAergic transmission.

3.3 Stress Increases $[^{35}S]TBPS$ Binding: Antagonism by Abecarnil

It is generally accepted that GABAergic transmission plays a major role in the changes of the emotional state and fear induced by environmental stimuli (see Biggio et al. 1990). Accordingly, different stressful conditions reduce the function of the $GABA_A$-receptor complex. This effect is similar to that elicited by inverse agonists of the benzodiazepine recognition site, tetrazol, and other negative modulators of GABAergic transmission which are known to elicit proconflict behavior in rat, experimental anxiety in monkey, and severe anxiety attack in man (see for review Biggio and Costa 1986). On the other hand, anxiolytic benzodiazepines, which enhance the function of GABAergic synapses in the mammalian central nervous system, elicit an opposite effect.

As expected from previous experiments (Concas et al. 1988; Serra et al. 1991), foot-shock stress increased the binding of $[^{35}S]TBPS$ in the rat cerebral cortex, an effect prevented by diazepam and alprazolam. Table 4 shows that abecarnil (0.5 mg/kg i.p.) administered to rats 30 min before foot-shock completely antagonized the increase in $[^{35}S]TBPS$ binding induced by this stressful stimulus.

This finding, consistent with other behavioral, pharmacological, and biochemical tests (Stephens et al. 1990), suggests that abecarnil, like other anxiolytic and antipanic compounds able to enhance the GABAergic transmission, had a marked effect in antagonizing the action of stress. These results indicate that the $GABA_A$–receptor complex plays a major role in the antistress effect of abecarnil.

3.4 CO_2 Inhalation Reduces $GABA_A$-Receptor Function: Antagonism by Abecarnil

To further investigate the anxiolytic and antistress action of abecarnil, we studied the effect of the drug on the reduction in GABAergic function

Table 4. Foot-shock stress enhances [^{35}S]TBPS binding in the rat cerebral cortex: antagonism by abecarnil

Treatment	[^{35}S]TBPS binding (fmols/mg prot)
Control	48.7 ± 2.2
Abecarnil	37.0 ± 2.6*
Foot-shock	63.6 ± 4.7*
Foot-shock + Abecarnil	49.1 ± 1.8

In order to avoid the stress associated with killing, rats were habituated to the handling maneuvers that precede killing (Biggio and Costa 1983). Abecarnil (0.5 mg/kg i.p.) was administered and foot-shock (5 min) was delivered 25 and 5 min before death, respectively. Each value is the mean ± standard error of mean of four separate experiments.
*$p < 0.05$ vs. control (analysis of variance followed by Scheffe's test).

Table 5. CO_2 inhalation enhances [^{35}S]TBPS binding in the the rat cerebral cortex: antagonism by abecarnil

Treatment	[^{35}S]TBPS binding (fmols/mg prot)
Control	51.4 ± 3.0
CO_2	76.0 ± 5.2*
FG 7142	66.8 ± 4.7*
β-CCE	62.7 ± 0.8*
CO_2 + abecarnil	58.3 ± 7**
CO_2 + alprazolam	55.4 ± 8**

In order to avoid the stress associated with killing, rats were habituated to the new environment (hermetically closed box, handling maneuvers that precede killing; Sanna et al. 1992). Rats were killed 10 min after 1 min exposure to CO_2; FG 7142 (12 mg/kg i.p.), β-CCE (25 mg/kg i.p.), abecarnil (1 mg/kg i.p.), and alprazolam (1 mg/kg i.p.) were administered 30 min before death. Each value is the mean ± standard error of mean of five separate experiments.
*$p < 0.05$ vs. control; **$p < 0.05$ vs. CO_2 (analysis of variance followed by Scheffe's test).

induced by CO_2 inhalation in the rat brain. We have recently found (Sanna et al. 1992; Concas et al. 1993) that in the brain of rats exposed to CO_2 inhalation, the stimulation of $^{36}Cl^-$ uptake induced by GABA was about 50% less than that found in the control, while the basal $^{36}Cl^-$ uptake was not modified by this treatment.

As expected from previous data (Sanna et al. 1992; Concas et al. 1993), the exposure of rats to CO_2 produced a significant increase in [^{35}S]TBPS binding in the rat cerebral cortex (Table 5). The effect of CO_2 on [^{35}S]TBPS binding was shared by β-carboline and FG 7142, two anxiogenic ligands for benzodiazepine recognition sites. Moreover, the effect of CO_2 was prevented by the administration of abecarnil and alprazolam. Consistent with the antagonistic action exerted on the foot-shock-induced increase in [^{35}S]TBPS binding (Table 4), the previous administration of abecarnil and alprazolam completely prevented the changes in the $GABA_A$-receptor function elicited by CO_2 inhalation.

The data reported demonstrate that abecarnil shares with alprazolam the ability to prevent the reduction in the function of $GABA_A$ ionophore–receptor complex elicited by a brief exposure of rats to CO_2 inhalation. Since the inhalation of carbon dioxide induces anxiety in healthy subjects and panic attack in patients with panic disorder (Woods et al. 1986), our finding suggests that a reduction in GABAergic transmission might be a major neurochemical event involved in the pharmacology and neurochemistry of carbon-dioxide-induced anxiety and panic attack. Such a conclusion would imply that abecarnil, like some benzodiazepines, has a potential antipanic action in man.

4 Failure of Chronic Abecarnil to Induce Tolerance and Dependence

It is well established that long-term treatment with benzodiazepines induces tolerance and physical dependence in mammals, including humans. Thus, several clinical studies have shown that the anticonvulsant, hypnotic, and anxiolytic effects of benzodiazepines may be altered by tolerance, and physical dependence may be detected by the presence of an abstinence syndrome upon the abrupt cessation of drug administration (Schopf 1983; Rickels et al. 1983; Murphy et al. 1984). Accordingly, the acute administration of flumazenil, a benzodiazepine recognition-site antagonist, to different animal species chronically treated with diazepam, precipitates a withdrawal syndrome characterized by the appearance of severe physical signs (Lukas and Griffiths 1982; Rosenberg and Chiu 1982).

4.1 Chronic Abecarnil in Mice

The ability of abecarnil to induce tolerance during long-term treatment was evaluated in mice using both behavioral (exploratory motility) and biochemical ([^{35}S]TBPS binding) parameters. We found that abecarnil, after acute i.p. administration, is very efficacious in reducing both the motor activity (Table 6) and the brain content of [^{35}S]TBPS binding (Table 6; Fig. 2) in this animal species.

To evaluate the neurochemical and behavioral aspects of tolerance, abecarnil (0.1 mg/kg i.p.) and diazepam (1 mg/kg i.p.) were administered chronically (three times daily for 2 weeks) at pharmacologically active doses to different groups of mice, and exploratory motility and cortical [^{35}S]TBPS binding were examined. In agreement with the literature (Gonsalves and Gallager 1987; Marley and Gallager 1989) chronic treatment with diazepam induced a marked reduction in the sensitivity of mice to this drug. In our

Table 6. Failure of abecarnil to induce tolerance in mice during chronic treatment

Abecarnil	Horizontal activity	[^{35}S]TBPS binding (fmols/mg prot)
Control + solvent	10 280 ± 1	26.1 ± 1.8
Control + abecarnil	1 336 ± 40*	18.3 ± 0.5*
Chronic treated + solvent	9 457 ± 472	22.4 ± 0.5
Chronic treated + abecarnil	3 598 ± 180**	15.6 ± 0.4**
Diazepam		
Control + solvent	10 535 ± 639	29 ± 7.2
Control + diazepam	4 740 ± 189*	21 ± 0.8*
Chronic treated + solvent	10 219 ± 204	32 ± 0.6
Chronic treated + diazepam	10 219 ± 306	31 ± 0.3

Data represent the mean ± standard error of mean of five separate experiments. Mice were treated with abecarnil (0.1 mg/kg i.p.) or diazepam (1 mg/kg i.p.) three times a day for 4 weeks. Controls were treated chronically with solvent. Mice were tested with a challenge dose (0.1 mg/kg abecarnil or 1 mg/kg diazepam). The motility was recorded 20 min after treatment. The test lasted 10 min, then the mice were killed and [^{35}S]TBPS binding performed.
*$p < 0.05$ vs. control + solvent; **$p < 0.05$ vs. chronic treated + solvent (analysis of variance followed by Scheffe's test).

study, as shown in Table 6, a challenge dose (1 mg/kg) of diazepam, markedly inhibited (60%–70%) exploratory motility in chronic solvent-treated animals, but failed to induce a significant change in the motor behavior of mice chronically treated with diazepam. Consistent with this behavioral effect, diazepam failed to reduce significantly the binding of [^{35}S]TBPS in the cerebral cortex of these chronic-treated animals, while markedly (−25%) reducing this binding in the brain of solvent-treated mice.

This finding clearly shows that long-term treatment with diazepam induces tolerance to the pharmacological efficacy of this drug. In contrast, in mice chronically treated with abecarnil the challenge dose (0.1 mg/kg) of this drug induced a marked reduction in both exploratory motility and [^{35}S] TBPS binding, an effect similar to that elicited in chronic solvent-treated mice by an acute administration of abecarnil. Table 6 shows that abecarnil was able to reduce, by about the same extent, the behavioral and the neurochemical parameters both in chronic abecarnil-treated mice and in solvent-treated animals.

The present finding indicates that abecarnil, a new anxiolytic and anticonvulsant ligand for benzodiazepine recognition site, failed to induce tolerance in mice during long-term treatment. In fact, although this drug was administered frequently (three times daily) and for a long time (4 weeks) in a pharmacologically efficacious dose, tolerance failed to occur during the treatment. This result is consistent with the atypical profile of this drug as compared to the classical benzodiazepines. Accordingly, although abecarnil shares with the latter drugs the anxiolytic and anticonvulsant action, together with the ability of enhancing the GABAergic function with high efficacy, this drug does not share with benzodiazepines the property to downregulate GABAergic transmission in responce to chronic treatment exposure.

This finding is consistent with the evidence that abecarnil fails to induce most of the side effects (clear signs of dependence, sedation, muscle relaxation, ataxia, etc.) common to benzodiazepines.

4.2 Chronic Abecarnil in Cats

Our and other laboratories have shown that cats are very sensitive to the acute and chronic action of benzodiazepine recognition-site ligands (Ongini et al. 1985; Giorgi et al. 1989). Accordingly within a few minutes of the acute administration of diazepam, severe motor incoordination associated with reduced muscle tone, marked ataxia, and sedation was induced in these animals. Moreover, in long-term treated animals tolerance rapidly developed to the above effects and the acute administration of flumazenil precipitated a dramatic withdrawal syndrome.

On the basis of this evidence we decided to compare the effect of chronic administration of diazepam and abecarnil in cats. The animals were treated i.p. three times daily with 7 mg/kg for 2 weeks with diazepam or abecarnil. As expected, the first doses of diazepam elicited the typical signs described above (Table 6). In contrast, abecarnil failed to induce these effects, cats treated with this compound showing only an evident alertness, a mild stimulatory effect, and increased voraciousness.

As shown in Table 7, 12 h after diazepam was last administered, the acute injection of flumazenil precipitated a severe withdrawal syndrome characterized by the appearance of severe physical signs. Within a few

Table 7. Effect of the acute administration of abecarnil and diazepam in the cat

	Abecarnil ($n = 6$)	Diazepam ($n = 4$)
Sedation	− − −	+ + +
Muscle Relazation	− − −	+ + +
Ataxia	+	+ + +
Alertness	+ + +	− − −
Aggressiveness (vs. mouse)	+ +	− − −
Fear (vs. mouse)	− − −	+ + +
Food intake	+ + +	+
Voraciousness	+ + +	+

One group of six cats and one of four were treated with abecarnil or diazepam (7 mg/kg i.p.) and observed for 4 hours

Table 8. Failure of flumazenil to precipitate a withdrawal syndrome in cats chronically treated with abecarnil

Withdrawal signs	Abecarnil ($n = 6$)	Diazepam ($n = 4$)
Tremors	– –	+ +
Increased muscle tone	– –	+ + +
Irritability	– –	– –
Fear	+	+ + +
Pupillary dilation	+ +	+ + +
Salivation	– –	+ +
Vocalization	– –	+ +

One group of six cats and one of four were treated with abecarnil and diazepam (7 mg/kg i.p. three times a day) for 15 days, respectively. Twelve hours after the last injection, 20 mg/kg flumazenil was administered i.p. and cats were observed until withdrawal signs were no longer present

minutes all the cats displayed tremors, increased muscle tone, repeated vocalizations, and salivation. Subsequently, they behaved frightened and rapidly withdrew to the back of their cages when attempts were made to remove them. In contrast, in all cats chronically treated with abecarnil, the i.p. administration of flumazenil failed to precipitate a clear abstinence syndrome. In fact, none of the abstinence signs present in diazepam-treated cats were observed in abecarnil-treated animals. Pupillary dilatation and mild fear were the only signs present 15–30 min after flumazenil administration. These effects lasted for not more than 60 min (Table 8).

Our data have shown that a sudden interruption in the chronic administration with the β-carboline derivative abecarnil is not associated with the discontinuation syndrome elicited by long-term treatment with benzodiazepines. Thus, although abecarnil is a benzodiazepine recognition-site ligand able to enhance the function of the GABA-coupled chloride channel with an efficacy similar or even greater than diazepam, it failed to share with the latter drug the ability to induce physical dependence in cats (see also Löscher et al., Sannerud et al., this volume).

This finding strongly suggests that in some experimental models abecarnil has a pharmacological profile typical of the partial agonist. Accordingly, it has been reported that flumazenil failed to precipitate withdrawal symptoms (Haefely et al. 1990) in squirrel monkeys chronically treated with high doses of the partial agonist bretazenil.

Finally, the failure of abecarnil to induce physical dependence can be considered consistent with the lack of this drug to enhance [^{35}S]TBPS binding in well-washed membranes. All together these results further suggest that abecarnil is devoid of some of the negative effects typical of benzodiazepines.

5 Conclusions

The present data suggest that the anxioselective and anticonvulsant abecarnil enhances the function of GABAergic synapses with an efficacy similar to diazepam, a benzodiazepine receptor full agonist, and much greater than that of the partial agonist bretazenil. These findings indicate that abecarnil can be considered a full, rather than a partial agonist at certain $GABA_A$ receptors.

However, the classification of abecarnil as a full agonist seems not to be in line with the findings reported in Tables 2, 6, and 7, and with previous studies suggesting that the drug is a partial agonist at central benzodiazepine receptors (Stephens et al. 1990; Turski et al. 1990; Löscher et al. 1990). Accordingly, despite its high potency and efficacy in antagonizing isoniazid-induced convulsions and reducing [^{35}S]TBPS binding in rat and mouse brain, low but pharmacologically active doses of the drug failed to induce motor impairment and induced only a slight sedation, and very high doses impaired motor coordination, leaving the righting reflex unaltered. Moreover, in mice and cats long-term treatment with abecarnil failed to induce tolerance and clear signs of dependence, two typical effects elicited by the chronic administration of benzodiazepines.

As a whole these experimental results suggest that abecarnil may act as a full agonist at benzodiazepine recognition sites coupled to those $GABA_A$ receptors mainly involved in anxiolytic and anticonvulsant action, and as a partial agonist at other subpopulations of receptors probably involved in the induction of some side effects.

This conclusion is consistent with the existence of multiple subpopulations of $GABA_A$/benzodiazepine receptors in the mammalian brain (Luddens and Wisden 1991). Thus, some specific pharmacological effects of abecarnil might be mediated by a selective activation of such different receptor subtypes in distinct brain areas.

In agreement with this idea, Pribilla et al. (this volume) have presented preliminary evidence that in frog oocytes-expressed $GABA_A$ receptors made up of α, β, and γ subunits, abecarnil shows much greater selectivity and potency at α_1-containing receptor subtypes than at α_3-containing subtypes.

In conclusion, abecarnil seems to be a new and more specific potential therapeutic agent for anxiety and seizures and also a new suitable tool to investigate the physiological and pharmacological role of $GABA_A$/benzodiazepine-receptor subpopulations in the mammalian brain.

Acknowledgments. This study was supported by grant 91.00087.PF41 from the National Research Council (CNR) – targeted project "Prevention and Control Disease Factors"; Subproject "Stress."

References

Biggio G, Costa E (eds) (1983) Benzodiazepine recognition-site ligands: biochemistry and pharmacology. Raven, New York

Biggio G, Costa E (eds) (1986) GABAergic transmission and anxiety. Adv Biochem Psych 41

Biggio G, Costa E (eds) (1990) GABA- and benzodiazepine-receptor subtypes. Adv Biochem Psych 46

Biggio G, Brodie BB, Guidotti A, Costa E (1977) Mechanism by which diazepam, muscimol and other drugs change the content of cyclic GMP in cerebellar cortex. Proc Natl Acad Sci USA 74:3592–3596

Biggio G, Concas A, Serra M, Salis M, Corda MG, Nurchi V, Crisponi C, Gessa GL (1984) Stress and β-carbolines decrease the density of low affinity GABA binding: an effect reversed by diazepam. Brain Res 305:13–18

Biggio G, Concas A, Corda MG, Serra M (1989) Enhancement of GABAergic transmission by zolpidem, an imidazopyridine with preferential affinity for type I benzodiazepine receptors. Eur J Pharmacol 161:173–180

Biggio G, Concas A, Corda MG, Giorgi O, Sanna E, Serra M (1990) GABAergic and dopaminergic transmission in the rat cerebral cortex: effect of stress, anxiolytic and anxiogenic drugs. Pharmacol Ther 48:121–142

Biggio G, Concas A, Costa E (eds) (1992) GABAergic synaptic transmission molecular, pharmacological and clinical aspects. Adv Biochem Psych 47

Concas A, Serra M, Atsoggiu T, Biggio G (1988) Foot-shock stress and anxiogenic β-carbolines increase t-[^{35}S]butylbicyclophosphorothionate binding in the rat cerebral cortex, an effect opposite to anxiolytics and γ-aminobutyric acid mimetics. J Neurochem 51:1868–1876

Concas A, Sanna E, Mascia MP, Serra M, Biggio G (1990) Diazepam enhances bicuculline-induced increase of [^{35}S]TBPS binding in unwashed membrane preparations from rat cerebral cortex. Neurosci Lett 112:87–91

Concas A, Mascia MP, Sanna E, Santoro G, Serra M, Biggio G (1991) "in vivo" administration of valproate decreases t-[^{35}S]butylbicyclophosphorothionate binding in the rat brain. Naunyn Schmiede bergs Arch Pharmacol 343:269–300

Concas A, Sanna E, Cuccheddu T, Mascia MP, Santoro G, Maciocco E, Biggio G (1993) Carbon dioxide inhalation, stress and anxiogenic drugs reduce the function of GAB$_A$-receptor complex in the rat brain. Prog Neuropsychopharmacol Biol Psychiatry 17 (in press)

Corda MG, Giorgi O, Longoni B, Ongini E, Montaldo S, Biggio G (1988) Preferential affinity of [^{3}H]2-oxo-quazepam for type I benzodiazepine recognition sites in the human brain. Life Sci 42:189–197

Gallager DW (1978) Benzodiazepines: potentiation of a GABA inhibitory response in the dorsal raphe nucleus. Eur J Pharmacol 49:133–143

Gee KW, Lawrence LJ, Yamamura HJ (1986) Modulation of the chloride ionophore by benzodiazepine-receptor ligands: influence of γ-aminobutyric acid and ligand efficacy. Mol Pharmacol 30:218–225

Giorgi O, Corda MG, Fernandez A, Biggio G (1989) The β-carboline derivative ZK 93426 and FG 7142 fail to precipitate abstinence signs in diazepam-dependent cats. Pharmacol Biochem Behav 32:671–675

Gonsalves SF, Gallanger DW (1987) Timecourse for development of anticonvulsant tolerance and GABAergic subsensitivity after chronic diazepam. Brain Res 405:94

Greenblatt DJ, Shader RI (1976) Benzodiazepines in clinical pracitice. Raven, New York

Haefely W (1984) Pharmacological profile of two benzodiazepine partial agonists: Ro 16-6028 and Ro 17-1812. Clinical Neuropharmacol 7 [Suppl 1]:670–671 (abstract S363)

Haefely W, Martin JR, Schoch P (1990) Novel anxiolytics that act as partial agonists of benzodiazepine receptors. TIPS 11:452–456

Horton WR (1980) GABA and seizure induced by inhibitors of glutamic acid decarboxylase. Brain Res Bull 5:605–608

Horton WR, Chapman AG, Meldrum BS (1979) Isoniazid, as a glutamic acid decarboxylase inhibitor. J Neurochem 33:745–750

Löscher W, Honack D, Scherke R, Hashem A, Frey HH (1990) Pharmacokinetics, anticonvulsant efficacy and adverse effects of the β-carboline abecarnil, a novel ligand for benzodiazepine receptors, after acute and chronic administration in dogs. J Pharmacol Exp Ther 255:541–548

Luddens H, Wisden W (1991) Function and pharmacology of multiple $GABA_A$-receptor subunits. TIPS 12:49–51

Lukas SE, Griffiths RR (1982) Precipitated withdrawal by benzodiazepine-receptor antagonist (Ro 15-1788) after 7 days of diazepam. Science 217:1161–1163

Marley RJ, Gallanger DW (1989) Chronic diazepam treatment produces regionally specific changes in GABA-stimulated chloride influx. Eur J Pharmacol 159:217–223

Murphy SM, Owen RT, Tyrer PJ (1984) Withdrawal symptoms after six weeks treatment with diazepam. Lancet 2:1389

Ongini E, Marzanatti M, Bamonte F, Monopoli A, Guzzon V (1985) A β-carboline antagonizes benzodiazepine actions but does not precipitate the abstinence syndrome in cats. Psychopharmacology (Berlin) 86:132–136

Polc P, Haefely W (1976) Effects of two benzodiazepines, phenobarbitone and baclofen on synaptic transmission in the cat cuneate nucleus. Naunyn Schmiedebergs Arch Pharmacol 294:121–131

Pritchett DB, Seeburg PH (1990) γ-aminobutyric $acid_A$ receptor $α_5$-subunit creates novel type II benzodiazepine receptor pharmacology. J Neurochem 54:1802–1804

Pritchett DB, Sontheimer H, Shivers BD, Ymer S, Kettenmann H, Schofield PR, Seeburg PH (1989a) Importance of a novel GABA-receptor subunit for benzodiazepine pharmacology. Nature 338:582–585

Pritchett DB, Luddens H, Seeburg PH (1989b) Type I and Type II $GABA_A$-benzodiazepine receptors produced in transfected cells. Science 245:1389–1392

Rickels K, Case WG, Downing RW, Winokur A (1983) A long-term diazepam therapy and clinical outcome. JAMA 250:767–771

Rosenberg HC, Chiu TH (1982) An antagonist-induced benzodiazepine abstinence syndrome. Eur J Pharmacol 81:153–157

Sanna E, Concas A, Serra M, Santoro G, Biggio G (1991) "ex vivo" binding of t-[^{35}S]butylbicyclophosphorotionate: a biochemical tool to study the pharmacology of ethanol at the γ-aminobutyric acid-coupled chloride channel. J Pharmacol Exp Ther 256:922–928

Sanna E, Cuccheddu T, Serra M, Concas A, Biggio G (1992) Carbon dioxide inhalation reduces the function of $GABA_A$ receptors in the rat brain. Eur J Pharmacol (in press)

Schopf J (1983) Withdrawal phenomena after long-term administration of benzodiazepines: a review of recent investigations. Pharmacopsychiatry 16:1–8

Serra M, Sanna E, Biggio G (1989) Isoniazid, an inhibitor of GABAergic transmission, enhances [^{35}S]TBPS binding in rat cerebral cortex. Eur J Pharmacol 164:385–388

Serra M, Sanna E, Concas A, Foddi MC, Biggio G (1991) Foot-shock stress enhances the increase of [^{35}S]TBPS binding in the rat cerebral cortex and the convulsions induced by isoniazid. Neurochem Res 16:17–22

Skerrit JH, Willow M, Johnston GAR (1982) Diazepam enhancement of low affinity GABA binding to rat brain membranes. Neurosci Lett 29:63–66

Squires RF, Casida JE, Richardson M, Saederup E (1983) ^{35}S-t-butylbicyclophosphorotionate binds with high affinity to brain-specific sites coupled to γ-aminobutyric $acid_A$ and ion recognition sites. Mol Pharmacol 23:326–336

Stephens DN, Schneider HH, Kehr W, Andrews JS, Rettig KJ, Turski L, Schmiechen R, Turner JD, Jensen LH, Petersen EN, Honore' T, Bondo Hansen J (1990) Abecarnil, a metabolically stable, anxioselective β-carboline acting at benzodiazepine receptors. J Pharmacol Exp Ther 253:334–343

Supavilai P, Karobath M (1984) t-butylbicyclophosphorotionate binding sites are constituents of the γ-aminobutyric acid benzodiazepine-receptor complex. J Neurosci 4:1193–1200

Turski L, Stephens DN, Jensen LH, Petersen EN, Meldrum BS, Patel S, Bondo Hansen
    J, Löscher W, Schneider HH, Schmiechen R (1990) Anticonvulsant action of the β-
    carboline abecarnil: studies in rodents and baboon, papio papio. J Pharmacol Exp
    Ther 253:344–352
Woods SW, Charney DS, Loke J, Goodman WK, Redmond DE, Heninger GR (1986)
    Carbon dioxide sensitivity in panic anxiety. Arch Gen Psychiatry 43:900–909

Abecarnil: A Novel Anxiolytic with Mixed Full Agonist/Partial Agonist Properties in Animal Models of Anxiety and Sedation

D.N. STEPHENS, L. TURSKI, G.H. JONES, K.G. STEPPUHN, and
H.H. SCHNEIDER

1 Introduction

Although the benzodiazepines are without doubt the most effective agents currently available for the treatment of anxiety disorders, they possess a number of properties which limit their use or which give rise to problems on withdrawal. Thus, currently available benzodiazepine anxiolytics are sedative and muscle relaxant, induce memory impairment, increase the intoxicating potency of alcohol, may be subject to nontherapeutic use (abuse), and, following chronic use, may give rise to problems of dependence. For these reasons, it has been the aim of medicinal chemistry to synthesize compounds with the therapeutic strengths of the benzodiazepines, but avoiding their unwanted properties. Given the proven efficacy of anxiolytics acting at benzodiazepine receptors, an obvious approach is to seek compounds acting at this site, but which have been modified so that the unwanted properties of the benzodiazepines have been eliminated. In recent years, two approaches have been used to achieve a better dissociation of the effects of benzodiazepine-receptor ligands; the first entails the use of compounds acting at partial agonists at benzodiazepine receptors (Haefely et al. 1990), but with the discovery of a number of subtypes of γ-amino-butyric acid type A (GABA$_A$) receptors, a second approach has become feasible. Although pharmacological evidence for benzodiazepine-receptor heterogeneity has existed for some time (Corda et al. 1988; Squires et al. 1979), it is only recently that the application of molecular biological techniques to the understanding of GABA$_A$ receptors has allowed us a fuller understanding of their complexity (see Lüddens, this volume). This approach, together with the heterogeneous distribution of the subtypes of GABA$_A$ receptors (see Turner, this volume), allows the hope that compounds acting selectively at GABA$_A$/benzodiazepine-receptor subtypes may also show selective aspects of the familiar benzodiazepine pharmacology.

The β-carboline substance class appears to offer potential for both approaches. Since the discovery that β-carboline-3-carboxylic acid ethyl ester (β-CCE) binds with high affinity to central benzodiazepine receptors

Research Laboratories of Schering AG, 13342 Berlin, Germany

(Nielsen and Braestrup 1980; see Braestrup and Nielsen, this volume), it has been demonstrated that structural derivatives may possess properties ranging from full inverse agonist to full agonist (Stephens et al. 1987). This range contains a number of partial agonists displaying anxiolytic and anticonvulsant properties differentiated from sedative and ataxic side effects (Petersen et al. 1984; Stephens et al. 1987). On the other hand, it has been known for some years that representatives of the β-carboline class show a preferential affinity for benzodiazepine type I (BZI) receptors in cerebellum (e.g., Poitier et al. 1988). This finding has been extended by the molecular biological approach to show, for instance, that β-carboline-3-carboxylic acid methyl ester (β-CCM) possesses a preference for α_1-containing receptors over α_2- or α_3-containing recombinants (Pritchett et al. 1989). This chapter will describe aspects of the pharmacology of a novel β-carboline, abecarnil, which achieves a selective pharmacological profile, partly through a selectively high affinity for certain receptor subtypes, and partly through a partial agonist action at some subtypes, and a full agonist profile at others.

2 Pharmacology of Abecarnil

Abecarnil is a β-carboline derivative which binds to the modulatory site of central $GABA_A$ receptors at which benzodiazepines also act (the so-called benzodiazepine receptor). Figure 1 illustrates the ability of abecarnil to displace ^3H-diazepam from membranes prepared from rat cerebral cortex with an affinity about 70 times higher than that of diazepam. Through its action at these sites, abecarnil possesses anxiolytic properties in a wide range of animal models, as listed in Table 1. These models include the classical conflict models in rodents, in which putative anxiolytics acting at 5-HT_{1A} or 5-HT_3 receptors are largely inactive, as well as ethologically derived models in monkeys and rodents. In rodent models, abecarnil is active at doses less than 0.5 mg/kg, reflecting a potency up to 100 times greater than that of diazepam. As is to be expected from anxiolytic compounds acting at central benzodiazepine receptors, abecarnil is also an effective anticonvulsant in a wide range of animal models (Turski et al. 1990).

In tests predictive of ataxic and muscle-relaxant properties of benzodiazepine-receptor ligands, however, abecarnil is either inactive even at high doses, or achieves its effects at doses some 30 times greater than those at which diazepam achieves the same effects (Table 2). This separation of the anxiolytic and ataxic properties of abecarnil is illustrated further in Fig. 2, in which the anxiolytic potencies of a series of benzodiazepine-receptor ligands, as well as other substances interacting with $GABA_A$ receptors, is plotted against their potency in a test of ataxia. The four-plate test (Boissier et al. 1968) is a simple test of anxiolytic activity, in which individual mice are

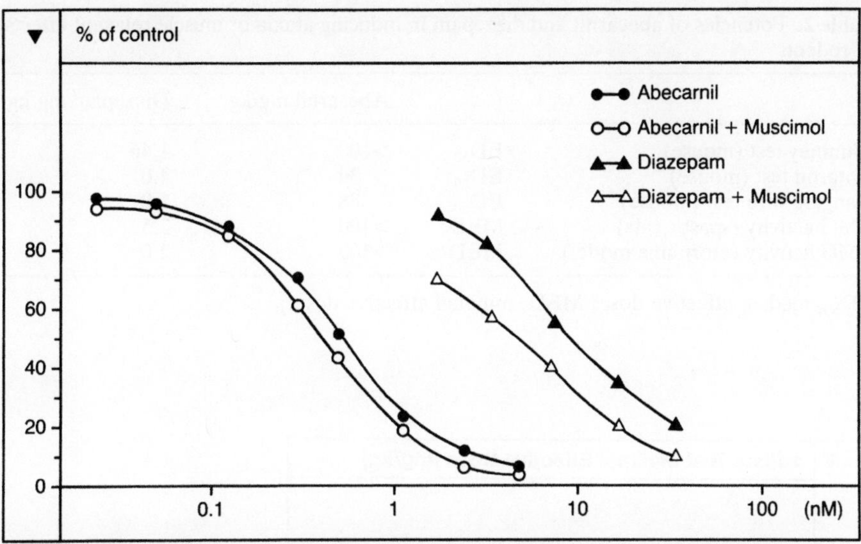

Fig. 1. Displacement by abecarnil and diazepam of ³H-diazepam binding from rat cerebral cortical membranes. Incubation was carried out at room temperature either in the presence of $50\,\mu M$ bicuculline (to ensure an absence of GABA), or in the presence of $30\,\mu M$ muscimol. Displacement of ³H-diazepam by diazepam was strongly enhanced in the presence of the GABA agonist by diazepam, and weakly enhanced by abecarnil

Table 1. Potency of abecarnil and diazepam in animal models predictive of anxiolytic activity

	Abecarnil mg/kg	Diazepam mg/kg	Source
Four-plate test (mouse) MED	0.1	0.39	Jones et al. 1993
Plus maze (mouse) MED	0.1	0.2	Jones et al. 1993
Operant conflict (rat)			
(Geller-Seifter type) MED	0.08	5.0	Stephens et al. 1990
Water-lick conflict (rat) MED	0.3	3.0	Stephens et al. 1990
Neophobia test (rat) MED	0.01	2.5	Fink et al., unpublished
Pentylenetetrazole cue (rat) ED_{50}	0.04	0.5	Stephens et al. 1990
Stress protection (rat) MED	0.3	1.0	Stephens et al. 1990
Monkey taming (cynomolgus) MED	10.0	10.0	Yamaguchi et al., unpublished

All values relate to effects following i.p. administration.
ED_{50}, median effective dose; MED, minimal effective dose.

allowed to explore a novel environment, but are punished with a weak electric shock when they cross certain divisions in the floor of the apparatus. This punishment results in a reduction in exploration, measured as the number of crossings of the floor divisions. In this simple conflict test, active

Table 2. Potencies of abecarnil and diazepam in inducing ataxia or muscle relaxant effects in rodents

		Abecarnil mg/kg	Diazepam mg/kg
Chimney test (mouse)	ED_{50}	>100	1.46
Rotarod test (mouse)	ED_{50}	30	4.0
Hanging wire test (mouse)	ED_{50}	38	1.0
EMG activity (spastic rats)	MED	>100	2.5
EMG activity (etorphine model)	MED	>100	2.0

ED_{50}, median effective dose; MED, minimal effective dose.

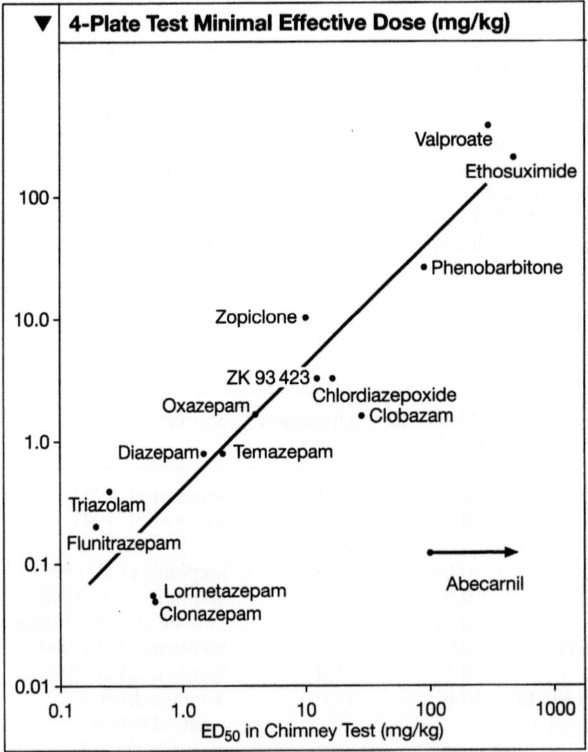

Fig. 2. Relationship of anxiolytic- and ataxia-inducing potencies in mice of substances acting at central $GABA_A$ receptors. Anxiolytic potency is expressed as the minimal effective dose in increasing activity suppressed by punishment in the four-plate test. Ataxic potency is the dose of drug which prevented 50% of mice from escaping from a vertical acrylic tube by climbing backwards to a height of 30 cm within 1 min

anxiolytics reinstate the exploratory activity which is suppressed by the punishment, in a dose-dependent manner. As a test of ataxia in the same species, the chimney test (Boissier et al. 1960) was chosen. In this test, mice are required to climb backwards up a narrow tube (chimney) in order to escape; substances which induce ataxia delay, or prevent the animals from climbing out of the tube. Figure 2 illustrates that the potencies in the two tests of a series of compounds acting at $GABA_A$ receptors are highly correlated. Abecarnil, however, falls off the regression line since it is a highly potent anxiolytic, but does not impair the abilities of the mice to escape from the chimney, i.e., has no ataxic properties in this model (Stephens et al. 1990).

Although abecarnil shows very weak activity in tests of ataxia and muscle coordination, its properties in tests of sedation are more complex (Stephens et al. 1990). In several tests predictive of sedation, abecarnil is considerably less potent than diazepam. Nevertheless, in other tests, particularly those in which the animal operates manipulanda for reward in operant chambers, abecarnil is markedly sedative. The reason for these apparent discrepancies between different measures of sedation is not known, but indicates that the term sedation covers several different qualities whose pharmacology is different.

3 Partial Agonism

This pattern of effects, potent anxiolytic activity combined with weak muscle-relaxant properties, is often attributed to a partial agonist profile of benzodiazepine-receptor ligands. Partial agonists are substances which, while binding to receptor sites with affinities similar to full agonists, are less efficaceous in achieving their action than full agonists. This phenomenon is well known in receptor pharmacology and is schematized in Fig. 3. In this figure, the abilities of three hypothetical benzodiazepine-receptor ligands to potentiate GABAergic transmission are shown. It is generally accepted that ligands for the modulatory site potentiate the effect of suboptimal concentrations of GABA, but the maximal GABA effect cannot be exceeded. Thus, for a given concentration of GABA, a full agonist will potentiate its effects to a maximum (within a given system) at doses giving rise to relatively low receptor occupancies (depending on receptor reserve). A compound with somewhat lower intrinsic efficacy will achieve the same maximal potentiation of GABA only at high levels of receptor occupancy, while a compound with even lower intrinsic activity will only partially potentiate the effects of GABA, even at doses giving rise to nearly full receptor occupancies. Of course, all degrees of partial agonism are possible between full and no effect.

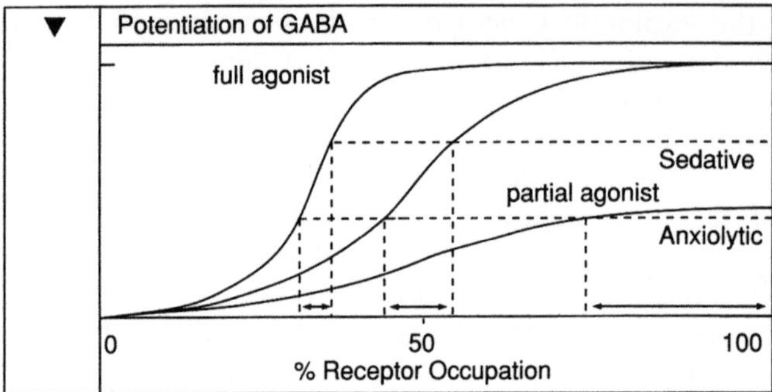

Fig. 3. Schematic diagram of the action of full and partial agonists at central benzo-diazepine receptors in potentiating the effects of GABA. According to experimental evidence, the different pharmacological effects of benzodiazepine-receptor ligands require different fractional receptor occupancies, and thus different levels of activation of GABAergic systems. The steepness of the response curve for full agonists determines that the separation of doses effective for anxiolysis and for sedation is poor; since partial agonists have a shallower dose–effect relationship in potentiating GABA, a better separation of pharmacological effects is observed, with weak partial agonists never achieving sufficient GABA facilitation to induce sedation, even at complete receptor occupancies

Within the assumption that benzodiazepine-receptor ligands produce similar effects at all of their receptors, these curves can then be used to generate certain predictions about the in vivo pharmacology of full and partial agonists. Thus, for instance, the dose–effect curves of full agonists should be steeper than for partial agonists, and they should achieve any given pharmacological end point at lower levels of receptor occupancy. Furthermore, it is known for conventional benzodiazepines that their sedative effects occur at higher doses (that is, higher levels of receptor occupancy) than their anxiolytic effects. This is illustrated in Fig. 3 as the sedative properties requiring a higher degree of GABA potentiation than the anxiolytic effects. In the scheme illustrated, the steepness of the slope of the receptor occupancy–effect curve for a full agonist leads to very narrow differences in the fractions of receptor occupancy (and also doses) at which its anxiolytic and sedative effects are reached. For less efficaceous compounds, with shallower receptor occupancy–effect curves, this "therapeutic window" is larger, while for weaker partial agonists, even at receptor occupancies approaching 100%, the potentiation of GABA may not be sufficient to induce sedation.

A great deal of our knowledge about the pharmacology of abecarnil can be explained through such a mechanism. Figure 1 shows that in binding studies, in vitro, in the absence of GABA, abecarnil displaces ^{3}H-diazepam from rat cerebellar membranes with an affinity about 70 times higher than that of diazepam itself. When the GABA$_A$ agonist, muscimol, is added to the incubation medium, the affinity of diazepam is increased 2.8-fold, consistent with diazepam, as a full agonist, showing a strong interaction with the binding of the GABA agonist. In contrast, the affinity of abecarnil for the same receptor site is only weakly (1.24-fold) influenced by the presence of the GABA agonist, consistent with a partial agonist action of abecarnil (Stephens et al. 1992).

In certain behavioral tests, too, abecarnil behaves in the way predicted for a partial agonist. From Fig. 3, it is clear that partial agonists need a higher fractional receptor occupancy than full agonists to achieve the same pharmacological effect. Figure 4 illustrates this phenomenon for the protection against pentylenetetrazole-induced convulsions in mice sensitized to the convulsant properties of pentylenetetrazole by repeated administration (kindling). Both diazepam and abecarnil were equally effective in their anticonvulsant action (Stephens et al. 1990), but, whereas diazepam protected all mice against seizures when occupying about 60% of receptors, abecarnil achieved the same effect only at a higher fractional receptor occupancy. A further example is seen in the case of the suppression of exploratory activity in Wistar rats exposed to a novel cage; whereas diazepam suppresses locomotor activity by 50% at a dose of 0.5 mg/kg, corresponding to a fractional receptor occupancy of about 12%, abecarnil achieves the same effect at 1.0 mg/kg, corresponding to a fractional receptor occupancy of 48% (Stephens et al. 1990).

A further prediction from the theory of partial agonism is that in those models in which partial agonists do not display sufficient efficacy to achieve the pharmacological end point, they should antagonize the effects of full agonists. For instance, in the chimney test of ataxia described above, abecarnil was inactive, but antagonized the ataxic effects of the benzodiazepine, lormetazepam (Stephens et al. 1990). Figure 5 illustrates the same phenomenon for a test of muscle relaxation (Turski and Stephens 1993). A mutant strain of the Wistar rat develops, during its development, a pathological

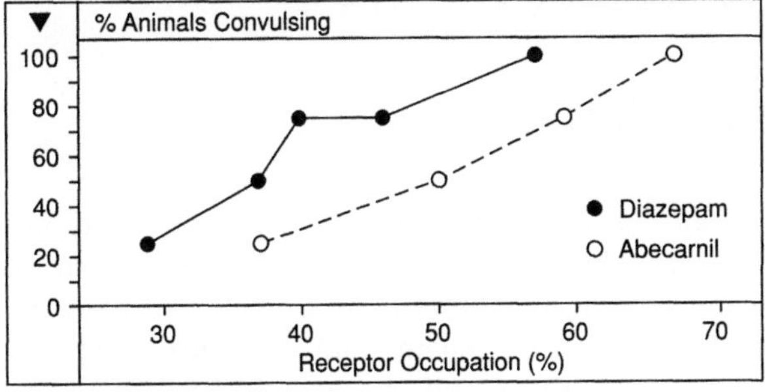

Fig. 4. Prevention of pentylenetetrazole-induced convulsions in kindled mice expressed as the elevation of the convulsant threshold induced by various doses of abecarnil or diazepam. The *ordinate* shows the fraction of ^{3}H-lormetazepam-labelled receptors occupied by the drug under investigation at the dose giving rise to the anticonvulsant effect. Abecarnil achieves its anxiolytic effect in this test at higher fractional receptor occupancies than diazepam, suggesting a partial agonist activity

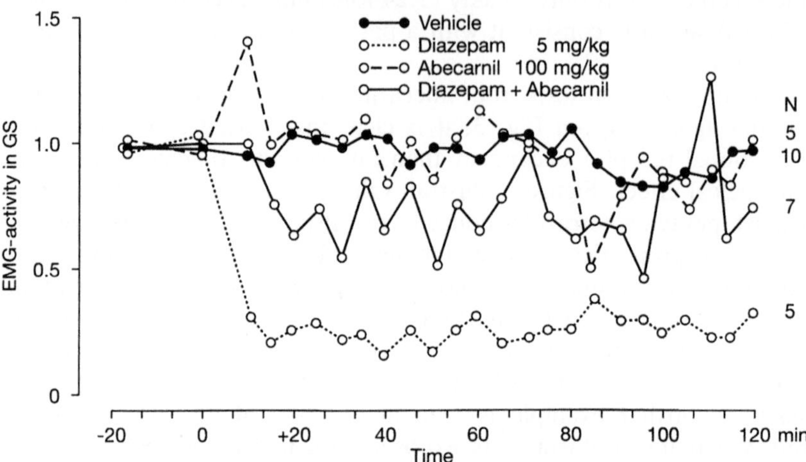

Fig. 5. Electromyographic (*EMG*) activity (normalized to 1) of the gastrocnemius (*GS*) muscle of spastic rats treated with vehicle ($n = 10$), with diazepam ($5\,mg/kg$, $n = 5$), or abecarnil ($100\,mg/kg$, $n = 5$), or a combination of the two drugs given i.p. ($n = 7$). The lack of activity of abecarnil itself in this test, combined with its ability to antagonize the muscle relaxant effect of diazepam, suggests a partial agonist activity in this model

increase in tone of extensor muscles of the hind limbs (Pittermann et al. 1976). This can be efficiently measured as increased electromyographic (EMG) activity, which is normalized by the administration of muscle relaxants, including benzodiazepines. While diazepam ($5\,mg/kg$, i.p.) reduces EMG activity of the spastic rat gastrocnemius muscle, abecarnil, even at doses as high as $100\,mg/kg$, possessed no muscle relaxant activity, but instead, antagonized the effect of diazepam. These findings are again consistent with abecarnil being a partial agonist at benzodiazepine receptors.

4 Full Agonism at Selective Receptors

Nevertheless, this latter result also suggests that partial agonism is not a complete explanation of the pharmacological properties of abecarnil. Studies of affinity for benzodiazepine receptors have shown that abecarnil possesses a much higher affinity than diazepam, and it is surprising that abecarnil antagonized the benzodiazepine only at such a high dose. This observation might suggest that at those receptors at which diazepam exerts its muscle relaxant action, abecarnil possesses a low affinity, consistent with a selectivity of abecarnil for receptor subtypes, as demonstrated in experiments with recombinant receptors (Pribilla et al., this volume; Knoflach et al. 1993).

Table 3. Ki values (nM) for the displacement of ^{3}H-flumazenil binding to rat brain membranes in GABA free conditions[a]

	Cerebellum	Spinal Cord
Diazepam	110 (3.3)	130 (4.4)
Abecarnil	0.24 (1.9)	1.3 (2.6)

[a] Values in brackets indicate GABA ratio values (ratio of Ki in GABA free condition to Ki in presence of GABA)

We have tested this possibility by studying the affinity of abecarnil for benzodiazepine receptors in spinal cord (where we assume benzodiazepines achieve their muscle-relaxant effects) and in the cerebellum, as representative of the central nervous system (CNS). Table 3 indicates that diazepam possesses a similar affinity for benzodiazepine receptors in the two regions, but that abecarnil has a fivefold higher affinity for cerebellar than for spinal-cord receptors. These findings suggest that abecarnil, indeed, has a lower affinity for the types of receptors found in spinal cord (principally receptors containing α_2 and α_3 subunits; see Turner et al., this volume). Is it possible, then, that part of abecarnil's selective pharmacological profile might be attributable to a selective action at certain subtypes of central $GABA_A$/-benzodiazepine receptors, as demonstrated for the recombinant receptor subtypes?

Figure 6 illustrates data from the lick-suppression test of anxiolytic activity in rats (Stephens et al. 1990), replotted in the form of fractional receptor occupancies obtained at doses used to obtain the antipunishment effect, as shown for the anticonvulsant data illustrated in Fig. 4. In contrast to the anticonvulsant data, however, in this test abecarnil achieves its antipunishment effect at levels of fractional receptor occupancy *lower* than those at which diazepam achieves comparable effects. This observation is *not* consistent with a partial agonist explanation, and suggests that abecarnil may be acting as a full agonist at a population of $GABA_A$ receptors responsible for the antipunishment properties of the drug. A similar effect was seen when abecarnil was compared with alprazolam in the four-plate test of anxiolytic activity (Fig. 7; Jones et al. 1993). In this figure, the anxiolytic effects of the two compounds are expressed as the percentage increase in punished locomotor activity on the abcissa, the ordinate showing the fractional receptor occupancies achieved at the drug dose used to induce the anxiolytic effect. The lower curve illustrates the changes in locomotor activity of independent groups of mice which were not punished, again expressed as a percentage of control values. In this experiment, alprazolam gave rise to a dose- (and hence receptor occupancy-) related increase in punished activity, reaching a 50% increase in activity at a receptor occupancy of about 20%. A similar antipunishment effect of abecarnil was seen at a

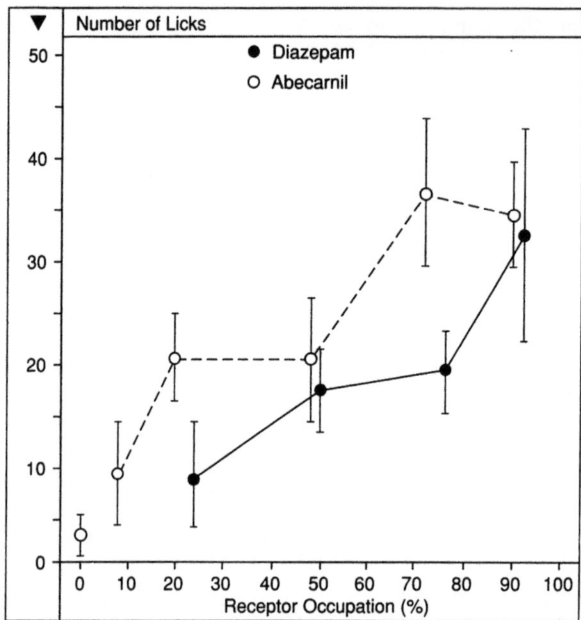

Fig. 6. Anxiolytic activity of abecarnil and diazepam measured as the elevation of the rate of punished licking by thirsty rats. The *ordinate* shows the fraction of ^{3}H-lormetazepam-labelled receptors occupied by the drug under investigation at the dose giving rise to the antipunishment effect. Abecarnil achieves its anxiolytic effect in this test at lower fractional receptor occupancies than diazepam, suggesting a full agonist activity

lower fractional receptor occupancy of less than 10%. The slope of the abecarnil curve was also steeper than that of alprazolam (cf. Fig. 2), though alprazolam appeared to give a somewhat greater relief of punishment-induced inhibition of activity. These results are again consistent with abecarnil possessing a similar, or even higher efficacy than alprazolam at the relevant receptor population for anxiolytic effects. Nevertheless, at higher levels of receptor occupancy, alprazolam became sedative, but abecarnil had no significant effects on unpunished activity, even at receptor occupancies approaching 100%, so that the effective anxiolytic dose range for abecarnil was much wider than that of alprazolam. Thus, although in a measure of anxiolytic potency abecarnil acted like a full agonist, in the measure of sedation the compound was ineffective, suggesting either that abecarnil has low affinity, or a low efficacy at the $GABA_A$/benzodiazepine-receptor population responsible for the sedative action of benzodiazepines in this test.

A full agonist type of action can be found in other tests of in vivo potency of the compound. For instance, blockade of $GABA_A$ receptors using the antagonist bicuculline can be overcome by using benzodiazepines to enhance the effects of GABA. Partial agonists are less effective in this

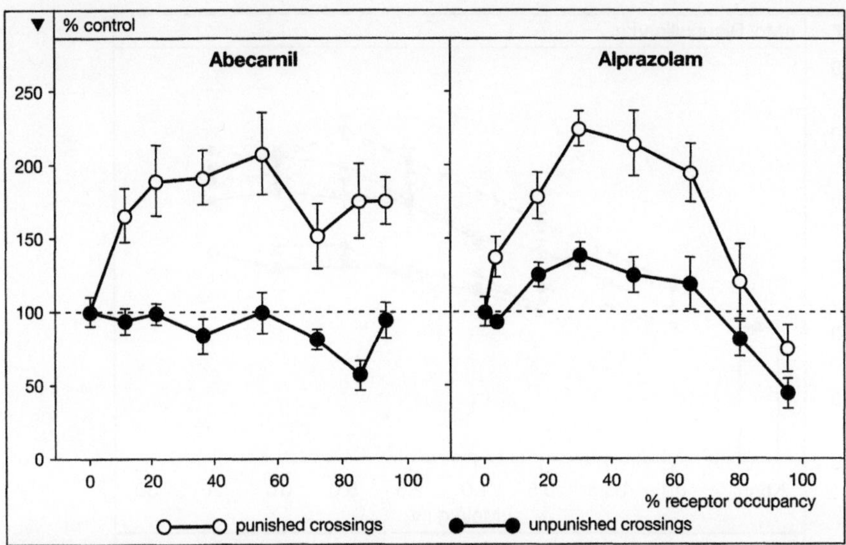

Fig. 7. Effects of abecarnil and alprazolam on punished and unpunished exploratory activity of independent groups of mice treated with various doses of the two drugs. Exploratory activity, measured as the number of crossings, is expressed as a percentage of the no-drug (vehicle) condition. In the unpunished condition this was approximately 13 crossings during the 1-min test and for the punished condition, five crossings. Drug doses are expressed as the fractional receptor occupancy reached by the dose tested, measured in vivo in parallel experiments using ^{3}H-lormetazepam as tracer. ○, punished crossings; ●, unpunished crossings

respect than full agonists. This phenomenon can be observed in vivo as the ability of benzodiazepines to elevate the convulsant threshold to bicuculline infused into the tail vein. Figure 8 shows the elevation in the bicuculline convulsion threshold induced by doses of several full and partial agonist compounds acting at benzodiazepine receptors (Stephens, unpublished). In this experiment, full benzodiazepine-receptor agonists, such as lorazepam and alprazolam, enhanced the convulsant threshold from 22 µmol/kg in control animals to a maximum of about 50 µmol/kg in the mice treated with the benzodiazepine. The maximal enhancement of convulsant threshold was similar for alprazolam and lorazepam, and was reached at drug doses giving rise to full receptor occupancies. In contrast to the full agonists, the benzodiazepine partial agonist, bretazenil, and the β-carboline partial agonist ZK 91296, elevated the convulsant threshold to only 30 µmol/kg, even at doses which gave rise to near complete receptor occupancy. Interestingly, in this model, alpidem resembled a partial agonist, whereas abecarnil achieved a maximal enhancement of convulsant threshold similar to that of the full agonists.

Overall, then, abecarnil shows a pharmacological profile characterized by potent anxiolytic-like qualities (Stephens et al. 1990; Jones et al. 1993),

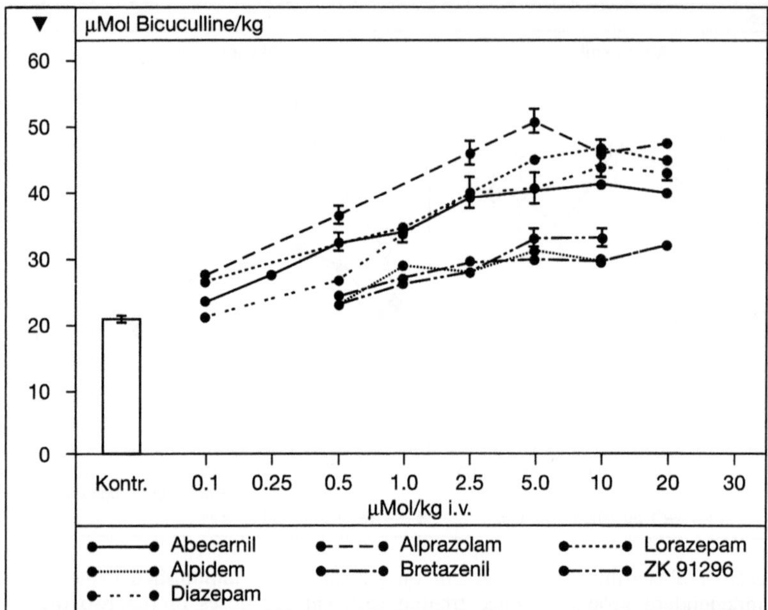

Fig. 8. Dose of intravenously applied bicuculline giving rise to the first clonic twitch during continuous infusion into the tail vein of mice, following treatment with vehicle, or with doses of benzodiazepine-receptor ligands administered i.v. 5 min before determination of the convulsant threshold. Note that drug doses are expressed in μmol/kg to facilitate comparisons of potencies

associated with anticonvulsant effects in a wide range of animal models (Turski et al. 1990; Löscher et al. 1990; Löscher and Hönack 1992; Crabbe 1992), but with few of the other properties, such as sedation and muscle relaxation common to conventional benzodiazepines. This differentiation of abecarnil's effects in vivo is partly attributable to a partial agonist activity at certain $GABA_A$/benzodiazepine receptor populations, but other aspects of abecarnil's pharmacology are best explained as being due to a full agonist action at other subtypes of $GABA_A$/benzodiazepine receptors. These in vivo results appear, then, to fit generally with observations obtained with recombinant $GABA_A$/benzodiazepine receptors, in which abecarnil acts as a full agonist at certain subunit combinations, but as a partial agonist at others (Pribilla et al., this volume; Knoflach et al. 1993), and with in vitro observations suggesting that abecarnil acts as a partial agonist in some brain tissues (Stephens et al. 1990), but as a full agonist at others (Serra et al., this volume). It must be emphasized, however, that it would be premature to associate a particular property of abecarnil in whole animal experiments, or in its clinical profile, with its action at particular subtypes of $GABA_A$ receptor. Suffice it to say that a mixed partial agonist/full agonist profile can be demonstrated at levels ranging from recombinant receptors, through in

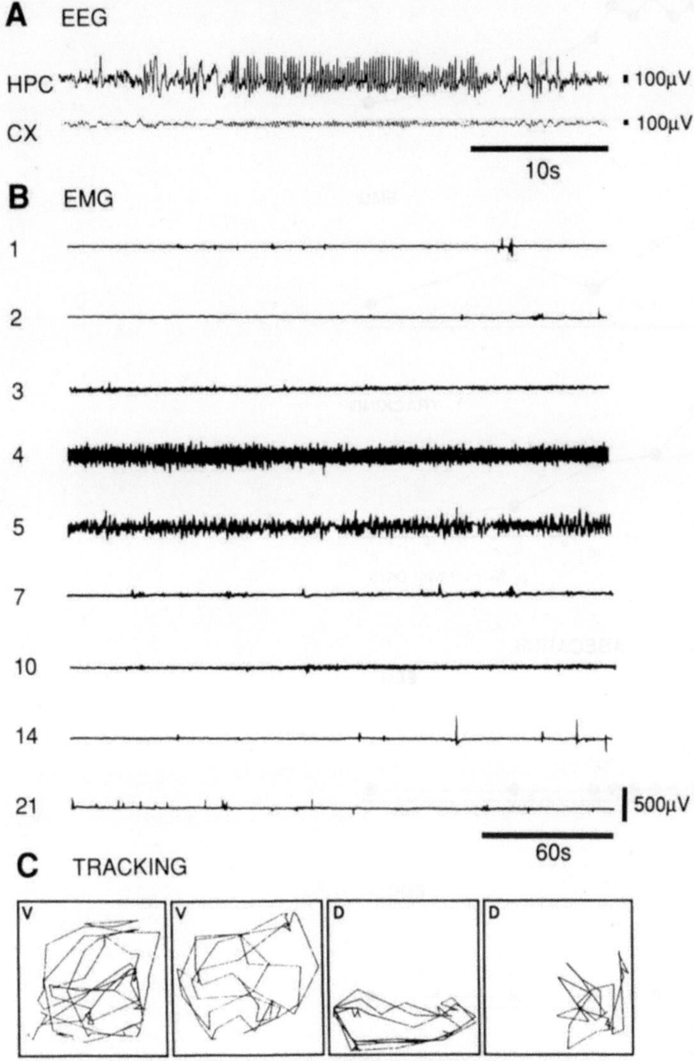

Fig. 9A–C. Original recordings of (**A**) electrographic seizures, (**B**) activity in gastro-cnemius muscle, and, (**C**) pattern of exploratory activity, in mice undergoing withdrawal from diazepam. **A** A typical seizure event recorded on withdrawal day 8 following 12 daily depot injections of diazepam (15 mg/kg); video recordings at this time showed gustatory automatisms and clonic movements of the forelimbs. **B** Temporal evolution of changes in the electromyograph (EMG) during withdrawal, showing enhanced myographic activity from day 4 of withdrawal. **C** Pattern of locomotor activity of individual mice exposed to a novel open field during withdrawal from vehicle (*V*) or diazepam (*D*) treatment, on withdrawal day 7. Note the thigmotaxic behavior of the mice in diazepam withdrawal, an indication of anxiety

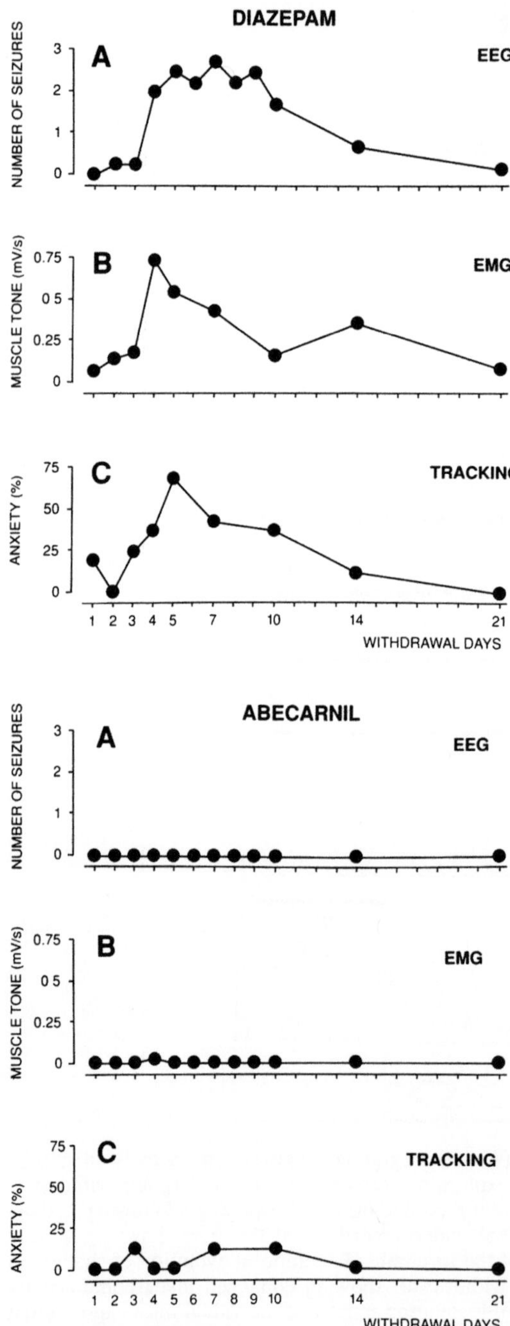

Fig. 10A–C. Time courses of (**A**) seizures, (**B**) changes in muscle tone, and (**C**) "anxiety" in mice during withdrawal from 12 days chronic treatment with diazepam (15 mg/kg daily as s.c. depot; *top panel*) or abecarnil (5 mg/kg; *bottom panel*)

vitro biochemical pharmacology of brain tissues, to its behavioral effects in a range of animal models.

5 Dependence Potential

It seems, then, that through its mixed action at $GABA_A$/benzodiazepine-receptor subtypes, abecarnil achieves a pharmacological profile of potent anxiolytic activity dissociated from muscle-relaxant and ataxic properties, and partially separated from sedative effects. How might the selective profile at receptor subtypes influence the dependence potential associated with benzodiazepines? This question will be addressed in detail in other chapters (see Sannerud et al., Löscher and Emmett-Oglesby et al., this volume), but it may be useful to describe here evidence obtained following chronic treatment of mice with abecarnil that the compound shows markedly less dependence potential than a conventional benzodiazepine.

Withdrawal of treatment from patients dependent on benzodiazepines results in a number of symptoms including anxiety, increased muscle tension, and rarely, but importantly, convulsions. These symptoms can be modelled in animals following withdrawal from chronic treatment with benzodiazepines. In our experiments, indwelling electrodes were used to continuously monitor seizure activity in cortex and hippocampus for 14 days following drug withdrawal; enhanced muscle tone was monitored by EMG measurements of spontaneous muscle activity, and changes in patterns of locomotor activity in an open field served as an indicator of anxiety (Steppuhn et al. 1993). Mice treated for 12 days with equipotent doses of diazepam (15 mg/kg) or abecarnil (5 mg/kg), given daily as a subcutaneous depot in sesame oil to ensure similar constant levels of receptor occupancy, were withdrawn from the drugs on day 12. Figure 9 illustrates examples of all three parameters measured during withdrawal from chronic treatment with diazepam. Epileptiform discharges were observed from withdrawal day 3 in most mice, as were increase in muscle tone and changes in the pattern of exploration of a novel open field, suggestive of increased anxiety. These observations are summarized in Fig. 10, which also shows that no such symptoms were seen in the mice withdrawn from abecarnil. These data show that it is possible to detect benzodiazepine withdrawal symptoms in mice, but that doses of abecarnil giving rise to a similar fractional receptor occupancy, and with similar kinetics, do not give rise to withdrawal symptoms.

6 Conclusions

The pharmacological profile of abecarnil, characterized by potent anxiolytic and anticonvulsant properties, combined with a lack of muscle relaxant effects, reduced sedation and interaction with ethanol, and markedly reduced dependence potential compared to benzodiazepines, reflects a complex interaction of the compound with $GABA_A$/benzodiazepine receptors. In many tests predictive of anxiolytic and anticonvulsant activity, the ability of abecarnil to achieve an effect at fractional receptor occupancies as low, or even lower than those of classical benzodiazepines, suggests a full agonist action. On the other hand, the lack of muscle-relaxant activity, the weak potentiation of ethanol (Stephens et al. 1990) and barbiturates (Turski et al. 1990), and weak sedative action in many tests is inconsistent with a uniformly high efficacy at all benzodiazepine receptors, while the compound's ability to antagonize the effects of benzodiazepines in models of ataxia and muscle relaxation is clear evidence of partial agonistic activity in those models. Although this pharmacological profile cannot at present be accounted for in detail, it is consistent with data from in vitro data on recombinant receptors indicating that abecarnil possesses full agonist activity at certain receptor combinations and partial agonist activity at others (Pribilla et al., this volume; Knoflach et al. 1993). Furthermore, this mixed full agonist/partial agonist profile at different receptor subtypes would also account for the observations of Serra et al., (this volume) of the high intrinsic efficacy of abecarnil in biochemical pharmacological measurements in vitro and in vivo, but a selective profile in vivo in behavioral models, and a lack of dependence potential.

References

Boissier JR, Tardy T, Diverres JC (1960) Une novelle methode simple pour explorer láction "tranquillisante": le test de la cheminee. Med Exp 3:81–84

Boissier JR, Simon P, Aron C (1969) A new method for the rapid screening of minor tranquillisers in mice. Eur J Pharmacol 4:142–150

Corda MG, Giorgi O, Longoni B, Ongini E, Montaldo S, Biggio G (1988) Preferential affinity of ^3H-2-oxoquazepam for type I benzodiazepine recognition sites in the human brain. Life Sci 42:189–197

Crabbe J (1992) Antagonism of ethanol withdrawal convulsions in Withdrawal Seizure Prone mice by diazepam and abecarnil. Eur J Pharmacol 221:85–90

Haefely W, Martin JR, Schoch P (1990) Novel anxiolytics that act as partial agonists at benzodiazepine receptors. Trends Pharmacol Sci 11:452–456

Jones GH, Schneider HH, Schneider C, Stephens DN (1993) Comparison of abecarnil with other benzodiazepine-receptor ligands in two models of anxiolytic activity in the mouse: an analysis based on fractional receptor occupancies. Psychopharmacology (in press)

Knoflach F, Drescher U, Scheurer L, Malherbe P, Möhler H (1993) Full and partial agonism displayed by benzodiazepine-receptor ligands at different recombinant $GABA_A$-receptor subtypes. Mol Pharmacol (in press)

Löscher W, Hönack D (1992) Withdrawal precipitation by benzodiazepine-receptor antagonists in dogs chronically treated with diazepam or the novel anxiolytic and anticonvulsant β-carboline abecarnil. Naunyn Schmiederbergs Arch Pharmacol 345:452–460

Löscher W, Hönack D, Scherkl R, Hashem A, Frey H-H (1990) Pharmacokinetics, anticonvulsant efficacy and adverse effects of the β-carboline, abecarnil, a novel ligand for benzodiazepine receptors, after acute and chronic administration in dogs. J Pharmacol Exp Ther 255:541–548

Nielsen M, Braestrip C (1980) Ethyl β-carboline-3-carboxylate shows differential benzodiazepine-receptor interaction. Nature 286:606–607

Petersen EN, Jensen LH, Honore T, Braestrup C, Kehr W, Stephens DN, Wachtel H, Seidelman D, Schmiechen R (1984) ZK 91296, a partial agonist at benzodiazepine receptors. Psychopharmacology 83:240–248

Pitterman W, Sontag K-H, Wand P, Rapp K, Deerberg F (1976) Spontaneous occurrence of spastic paresis in Han-Wistar rats Neurosci Lett 2:45–49

Poitier MC, Prado de Carvalho L, Dodd RH, Besselievre R, Rossier J (1988) In vivo binding of β-carbolines in mice: regional differences and correlation of occupancy to pharmacological effects. Mol Pharmacol 34:124–128

Pritchett DB, Lüddens H, Seeburg PH (1989) Type I and Type II GABA$_A$-benzodiazepine receptors produced in transfected cells. Science 245:1389–1392

Squires RF, Benson DI, Braestrup C, Coupet J, Klepner CA, Myers V, Beer B (1979) Some properties of brain-specific benzodiazepine receptors: new evidence for multiple receptors. Pharmacol Biochem Behav 10:825–830

Stephens DN, Schneider HH, Kehr W, Jensen LH, Petersen EN, Honore T (1987) Modulation of anxiety by β-carbolines and other benzodiazepine-receptor ligands: relationship of pharmacological to biochemical measures of efficacy. Brain Res Bull 19:309–318

Stephens DN, Schneider HH, Kehr W, Andrews JS, Rettig K-J, Turski L, Schmiechen R, Turner JD, Jensen LH, Petersen EN, Honore T, Bondo Hansen J (1990) Abecarnil, a metabolically stable, anxioselective β-carboline acting at benzodiazepine receptors. J Pharmacol Exp Ther 253:334–343

Stephens DN, Turski L, Hillman M, Turner JD, Schneider HH, Yamaguchi M (1992) What are the differences between abecarnil and conventional benzodiazepine anxiolytics? In: Biggio G, Concas A, Costa E (eds) GABAergic synaptic transmission. Raven, New York, pp 395–405

Steppuhn K, Schneider HH, Turski L, Stephens DN (1993) Long-term treatment with abecarnil does not lead to dependence in mice. J Pharmacol Exp Ther 264:1395–1400

Turski L, Stephens DN, Jensen LH, Petersen EN, Meldrum BS, Patel S, Bondo Hansen J, Löscher W, Schneider HH, Schmiechen R (1990) Anticonvulsant action of the β-carboline, abecarnil: studies in rodents and baboon, Papio papio. J Pharmacol Exp Ther 253:344–352

Turski L, Stephens DN (1993) Effects of the β-carboline, abecarnil, on spinal reflexes in mice, and on muscle tone in genetically spastic rats: a comparison with diazepam. J Pharmacol Exp Ther (in press)

Abecarnil Shows Reduced Tolerance Development and Dependence Potential in Comparison to Diazepam: Animal Studies

W. Löscher

1 Introduction

Development of tolerance and dependence limits the therapeutic use of traditional benzodiazepine-(BZ) receptor agonists, such as diazepam (Owen and Tyrer 1983; Woods et al. 1987; Haefely et al. 1990). Recent reports have indicated that partial (low efficacy) BZ-receptor agonists, i.e., compounds which induce smaller fractional responses in their target cells than do full agonists at the same fractional receptor occupancy, may have advantages in this respect, because low-efficacy agonism prevents overstimulation of a receptor population, thereby reducing overdose problems, desensitization responses, and adaptation (Haigh and Feely 1988; Haefely et al. 1990). Indeed, repeated treatment of mice with the partial BZ-receptor agonist, bretazenil (Ro 16-6028), produced no significant tolerance to the anticonvulsant effect, in contrast to the effect of full agonists (Haigh and Feely 1988). Furthermore, again unlike full agonists, physical dependence could not be induced in squirrel monkeys after repeated very high doses of bretazenil as assessed by challenge with the BZ-receptor antagonist, flumazenil (Haefely et al. 1990). Although these data on bretazenil indicate that partial BZ-receptor agonism might have important practical consequences, there are also studies on other partial BZ-receptor agonists reporting less favorable data. Thus, during chronic treatment of dogs with clonazepam, which has a lower intrinsic efficacy than diazepam (Haefely et al. 1990), there was only a slight reduction in anticonvulsant potency during chronic treatment, but severe withdrawal symptoms, including seizures, were seen upon abrupt termination of treatment (Scherkl et al. 1985; Scherkl and Frey 1986). Similarly, during chronic treatment of dogs with clorazepate, a prodrug of desmethyldiazepam, which acts as a partial agonist at BZ receptors (Frey and Löscher 1982; Gobbi et al. 1987), no tolerance developed to the anticonvulsant effect, but again severe withdrawal symptoms were observed

Department of Pharmacology, Toxicology, and Pharmacy, School of Veterinary Medicine, Bünteweg 17, 30559 Hanover 71, Germany upon discontinuation of treatment (Scherkl et al. 1989). This clearly demonstrates that during treatment with BZs that act as partial BZ-receptor agonists, physical dependence may occur without obvious tolerance. This apparent separation of BZ tolerance and dependence has also been demonstrated in rodents (Wilson et al. 1989).

More recently, the preclinical pharmacological properties of abecarnil, an anxiolytic and anticonvulsant β-carboline with high affinity for central BZ receptors, have been described (Stephens et al. 1990; Turski et al. 1990). Like bretazenil, abecarnil is effective in lower doses than diazepam in tests predictive of anxiolytic and antiepileptic activity, but is clearly less potent than diazepam in tests of sedation and muscle relaxation and even antagonizes the motor-impairing effects of traditional BZs, a pharmacological profile characteristic of partial BZ-receptor agonism (Stephens et al. 1990; Turski et al. 1990). However, there are certain features of the pharmacology of abecarnil which are less consistent with a partial agonist classification but suggest a preference of abecarnil for subtypes of a heterogeneous BZ-receptor population (Turski et al. 1990; Stephens et al. 1990, 1991).

Irrespective of whether abecarnil is a selective or a partial agonist at central BZ receptors, chronic experiments in rodents have indicated that abecarnil might have advantages over BZs with respect to development of tolerance. In mice, repeated treatment with abecarnil (15 mg/kg i.p., twice daily for 12 days) led to a slight reduction in its potency to increase the threshold for induction of clonic seizures by pentylenetetrazol (PTZ; Schneider et al. 1990). However, abecarnil remained to exert significant anticonvulsant effects throughout the period of treatment (Schneider et al. 1990), and the reduction in its anticonvulsant potency in the PTZ seizure-threshold model was much less marked compared to full BZ-receptor agonists, such as diazepam, in the same model (Haigh and Feely 1988). Similarly, using amygdala-kindled rats as a model of complex partial seizures, abecarnil showed reduced tolerance development in comparison to standard benzodiazepines, such as clobazam (Löscher and Rundfeldt 1990; Löscher et al. 1991).

In order to obtain more information on tolerance development during longterm treatment with abecarnil, we used dogs as a model. This species offers the advantage that in addition to tolerance the dependence potential of BZ-receptor ligands can be studied in more detail than in rodents. Indeed, as shown previously by different groups, withdrawal symptoms precipitated in dogs by abrupt termination of chronic BZ treatment or by administration of BZ-receptor antagonists are similar to those observed in humans (McNicholas et al. 1983; Scherkl et al. 1985; Scherkl and Frey 1986; Löscher et al. 1989; Scherkl et al. 1989). The data which were obtained with abecarnil and diazepam in dogs (Löscher et al. 1989, 1990; Löscher and Hönack 1992) will be described and discussed in the present paper.

2 Chronic Experiments with Abecarnil and Diazepam in Dogs

2.1 Alterations in Anticonvulsant Potency of Abecarnil During Chronic Administration and Effect of Flumazenil Injection

In order to allow a comparison with the chronic efficacy of diazepam, clonazepam, and clorazepate determined in previous experiments in dogs (Frey et al. 1984; Scherkl et al. 1985, 1989), a treatment protocol for abecarnil very similar to that used in the previous BZ studies was chosen, except that abecarnil was administered by the s.c. route for maintenance treatment between weekly PTZ threshold determination, while BZs had been administered orally. Previous experiments with abecarnil in dogs had shown that oral administration of abecarnil is unsuitable for maintenance treatment because of too low a bioavailability and too rapid an elimination of the β-carboline after this route of administration (Löscher et al. 1990). However, active drug concentrations can be maintained during chronic treatment by a daily s.c. injection of the drug suspended in peanut oil (Löscher et al. 1990). Indeed, when injected s.c. as a suspension in peanut oil, abecarnil is absorbed only slowly so that a daily injection results in an accumulation of plasma drug concentrations during chronic treatment.

Anticonvulsant potency of abecarnil was evaluated by determining the seizure threshold after i.v. infusion of PTZ as described previously (Löscher 1982, 1983; Frey et al. 1984; Scherkl et al. 1985, 1989). Results of experiments with chronic administration of abecarnil are shown in Fig. 1. Compared to the acute anticonvulsant potency of abecarnil determined after a single dose i.v. injection of 0.5 mg/kg before the onset of chronic treatment, anticonvulsant potency of the same i.v. dose was markedly increased after 1 week of treatment with a daily s.c. injection of the β-carboline. This might indicate that the drug had accumulated in the brain during daily s.c. administration, although plasma concentrations 10 min after administering abecarnil i.v., i.e., at the time of PTZ infusion, were about the same as before onset of chronic treatment (Fig. 1). Maximum anticonvulsant efficacy was determined after 1–2 weeks of treatment, but after further treatment a certain reduction in the effect on the PTZ threshold was observed in some dogs. However, the average seizure threshold remained far above control values throughout the period of treatment (Fig. 1). In a vehicle control experiment, PTZ seizure threshold remained at a constant level on all experimental days (not illustrated).

Plasma levels of abecarnil determined during and after the period of treatment at days of seizure-threshold determinations are shown in Fig. 1. During treatment, average plasma levels analyzed in the seven dogs remained relatively constant, although there was a tendency to increased levels in the fifth and sixth week of treatment. Trough levels measured before i.v. injection of abecarnil, i.e., concentrations of the β-carboline 24 h

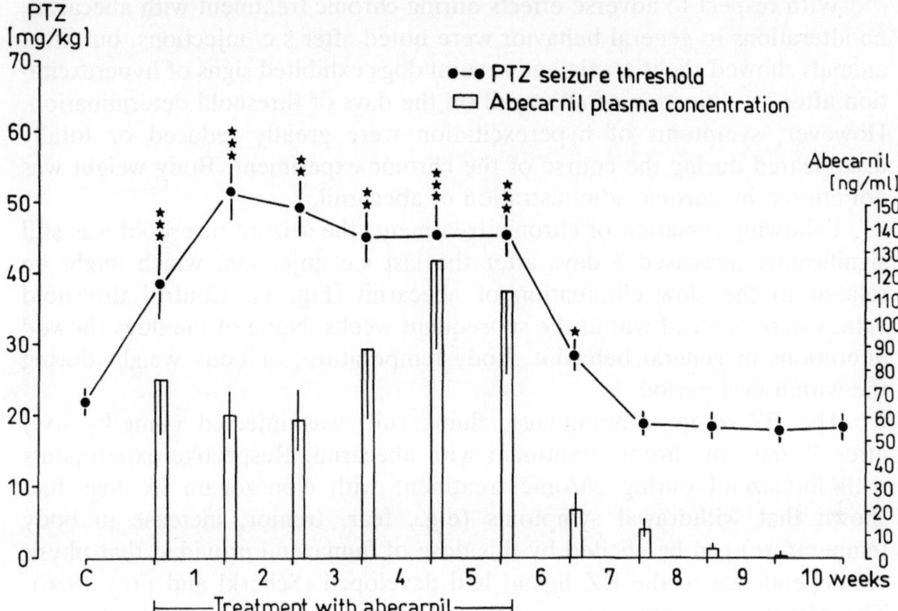

Fig. 1. PTZ seizure threshold in seven beagle dogs before, during, and after chronic treatment with abecarnil. Before onset of drug treatment, the control threshold was repeatedly determined at weekly intervals. Drug testing was not started before reproducible seizure thresholds were obtained in all animals. One week after determination of the last control seizure threshold, either vehicle (40% glycofurol in water) or 0.5 mg/kg abecarnil were injected i.v. and the threshold was determined 10 min thereafter. Chronic treatment was then started with a daily s.c. injection of 4 mg/kg abecarnil suspended in peanut oil. During chronic treatment, the PTZ threshold was determined once a week in the morning 10 min after i.v. injection of the β-carboline (0.5 mg/kg). On these days, s.c. injection of abecarnil was done in the afternoon, while on all other days the suspension was injected in the morning. Chronic treatment was terminated after 40 days and the PTZ threshold was determined at weekly intervals during the withdrawal period until stable control values were reached again. The PTZ seizure threshold is shown as means ± SE; significant differences from control threshold (calculated by the Wilcoxom signed ranks test for paired replicates) are indicated by asterisks (*$p < 0.05$; **$p < 0.02$; ***$p < 0.01$). The control threshold shown in the figure represents the mean ± SE of 35 determinations in the seven dogs used for chronic administration of the β-carboline. In addition to threshold data, the figure shows plasma concentrations (means ± SE) of abecarnil determined immediately prior to onset of PTZ infusion at days with seizure-threshold determinations

after the last s.c. injection, ranged between 10 and 19 ng/ml (not illustrated). Following cessation of chronic treatment, plasma levels slowly declined with an average half-life of 84 h (Fig. 1), thus demonstrating the very slow absorption of abecarnil from s.c. injection sites, which was also observed after acute single-dose injection of the drug in peanut oil (Löscher et al. 1990).

With respect to adverse effects during chronic treatment with abecarnil, no alterations in general behavior were noted after s.c. injections, but most animals showed slight ataxia and several dogs exhibited signs of hyperexcitation after i.v. injection of abecarnil on the days of threshold determination. However, symptoms of hyperexcitation were greatly reduced or totally disappeared during the course of the chronic experiment. Body weight was not altered by chronic administration of abecarnil.

Following cessation of chronic treatment, the seizure threshold was still significantly increased 3 days after the last s.c. injection, which might be related to the slow elimination of abecarnil (Fig. 1). Control threshold values were reached within the subsequent weeks. None of the dogs showed alterations in general behavior, body temperature, or body weight during the withdrawal period.

The BZ-receptor antagonist, flumazenil, was injected (1 mg/kg i.v.) after 38 days of chronic treatment with abecarnil. Respective experiments with flumazenil during chronic treatment with clonazepam in dogs had shown that withdrawal symptoms (e.g., fear, tremor, increase in body temperature) can be elicited by this dose of flumazenil provided that physical dependence to the BZ ligand had developed (Scherkl and Frey 1986). The plasma concentration of abecarnil in the seven dogs at the time of injection of the BZ-receptor antagonist (about 2 h after s.c. injection of abecarnil) was 23.5 ng/ml (range 8–58 ng/ml). Body temperature was not altered after injection of flumazenil. In two dogs, a slight tremor was observed after 40–50 min, other changes in general behavior were not seen. In three control dogs, flumazenil had no effect on body temperature or general behavior at the dosage administered.

2.2 Use of Different BZ-receptor Antagonists to Precipitate Withdrawal Signs After Chronic Treatment with Either Diazepam or Abecarnil

In further experiments, six dogs were treated chronically with diazepam or abecarnil with a cross-over design. Time intervals between the different chronic drug experiments in the same group of dogs were 3 months. For withdrawal precipitation by BZ-receptor antagonists, either flumazenil or the β-carboline ZK 93426 were given, using an i.v. infusion technique previously developed for withdrawal precipitation in diazepam-dependent rats and dogs (Wilson and Gallager 1988; Löscher et al. 1989). The rationale to use not only flumazenil but also a BZ-receptor antagonist with β-carboline structure (ZK 93426) was based on the possibility that BZs and β-carbolines bind, at least in part, to different subpopulations of the BZ receptor. Thus, in animals chronically treated with a β-carboline such as abecarnil, withdrawal signs precipitated by flumazenil might differ from those precipitated by a β-caboline antagonist.

For the testing of precipitated withdrawal, solutions of the BZ antagonists, flumazenil or ZK 93426 in 50% glycofurol, were infused i.v. at a constant rate (3 ml/min) up to a dose of 20 mg/kg. This technique of inducing withdrawal has been recently described by Wilson and Gallager (1988) for rats and by Löscher et al. (1989) for dogs. In order to differentiate withdrawal symptoms from effects induced by the BZ antagonists or the vehicle (50% glycofurol) used for solutions of antagonists, it was necessary to study the effects of vehicle and BZ antagonists in diazepam-naive dogs prior to onset of chronic treatment. The dose of antagonists chosen (20 mg/kg) corresponded to the maximum dose infused i.v. for withdrawal precipitation in diazepam-dependent rats by Wilson and Gallager (1988) and diazepam-dependent dogs by Löscher et al. (1989). For the evaluation of vehicle and antagonist effects, all six diazepam-naive dogs received vehicle infusion at the chosen rate and total volume and, 3–5 days later, infusion of vehicle plus antagonist (three dogs flumazenil and three dogs ZK 93426). The animals were closely examined for changes in general behavior during several hours after the infusion as described in detail elsewhere (Löscher et al. 1989).

2.2.1 Effects of BZ-Receptor Antagonists in Diazepam-Naive Dogs

In the acute experiments with i.v. infusion of BZ antagonists or vehicle alone in diazepam-naive dogs, it was found that at the infusion rate (3 ml/min) and maximum infusion volume (2 ml/kg) chosen, the glycofurol vehicle alone caused transient ataxia (slight weakness in hind legs for about 30–120 s after termination of infusion) in five of six dogs examined, and an increase in body temperature in two dogs. After infusion of flumazenil (20 mg/kg), ataxia was much more marked and of longer duration than ataxia observed with vehicle alone and the dogs showed sedation and vocalization, indicating that flumazenil exerted effects of its own. In contrast, ataxia occurring after infusion of ZK 93426 (20 mg/kg) was not different from that observed in the same dogs with vehicle alone, indicating that ZK 93426, at least in dogs, is a more neutral antagonist than is flumazenil.

2.2.2 Chronic Experiments with Diazepam

For the chronic experiments, doses and dosing intervals for diazepam were chosen on the basis of previous experiments in dogs (Löscher and Frey 1981; Frey et al. 1984). In all experiments with diazepam and abecarnil, those dogs which had received flumazenil or ZK 93426 in the acute experiments prior to chronic drug treatment received the same antagonist after chronic drug treatment to allow a direct comparison of effects.

Three times daily oral treatment of the animals with 1 mg/kg diazepam for 1 week did not cause any observable side effects, nor did it change body temperature or body weight. Plasma concentrations of diazepam and its metabolites during the period of treatment demonstrated that diazepam is extensively metabolized in dogs so that even after the first dose levels of desmethyldiazepam and oxazepam were several times higher than those of the parent drug. After repeated dosing, maximum drug and metabolite levels were higher than those determined after the first dosing with diazepam, indicating accumulation. However, even after accumulation, diazepam levels did not exceed 30 ng/ml, whereas maximum levels of oxazepam and desmethyldiazepam of about 100 and 400 ng/ml, respectively, were determined during prolonged diazepam treatment (not illustrated). Immediately before infusion of the BZ-receptor antagonists, i.e., 1 h after the last oral dosing with diazepam at day 7 of the trial, average levels of diazepam, oxazepam, and desmethyldiazepam were 8, 62, and 280 ng/ml, respectively. Infusion of flumazenil or ZK 93426 induced behavioral symptoms in some of the animals which were not present after injection of either vehicle or antagonist in diazepam-naive dogs, indicating that only 1 week of treatment with relatively low doses of diazepam had led to the development of physical dependence (Fig. 2). Thus, with flumazenil in one dog marked hyperexcitation was induced with generalized tremor, myoclonic jerks, hyperventilation, disturbed gait with retarded setting of paws, transient circling, and retching. A second dog showed generalized tremor, whereas the third dog tested with flumazenil did not exhibit abstinence symptoms. With ZK 93426, behavioral changes observed were less pronounced compared to flumazenil. One dog vomited, whereas a second dog showed twitches and jerks, mainly of the head. There were no marked changes in body temperature after infusion of the antagonists (Fig. 2). On the days after the last administration of diazepam, no further behavioral changes and no changes in body temperature or body weight were noted.

During three times daily oral treatment of dogs with 2 mg/kg diazepam for 2 weeks, diazepam did not cause any observable side effects nor did it change body temperature or body weight. As in the first trial, diazepam was extensively metabolized in the animals. Immediately prior to infusion of antagonists, i.e., 1 h after the last dose of diazepam at day 15 of the trial, average levels of diazepam, oxazepam, and desmethyldiazepam were 75, 67, and 1200 ng/ml, respectively. Infusion of antagonists precipitated marked withdrawal symptoms in all dogs tested, but differences were observed between the two antagonists (Fig. 2). With flumazenil, all three dogs showed hyperexcitation and/or generalized tremor during the i.v. infusion, which, however, was continued up to the maximum dose of 20 mg/kg. After the infusion, the dogs were immobile with rigid postures (two dogs in a prone position) and increased muscle tone in limbs (as determined by palpation), and exhibited generalized tremor, and twitches and jerks of head, limbs, or body. In addition, two dogs showed pronounced hyperventilation. Immobility lasted for 10–30 min, after which two of the animals still had a disturbed gait with retarded setting of paws and/or rigid walking. In one dog, transient circling was seen. Twitches and jerks were observed for up to 3 h after the infusion.

With ZK 93426, one dog exhibited tremor and two dogs myoclonic jerks during the last minute of infusion. After the infusion, in contrast to flumazenil the dogs were able to run around normally (although hot-foot

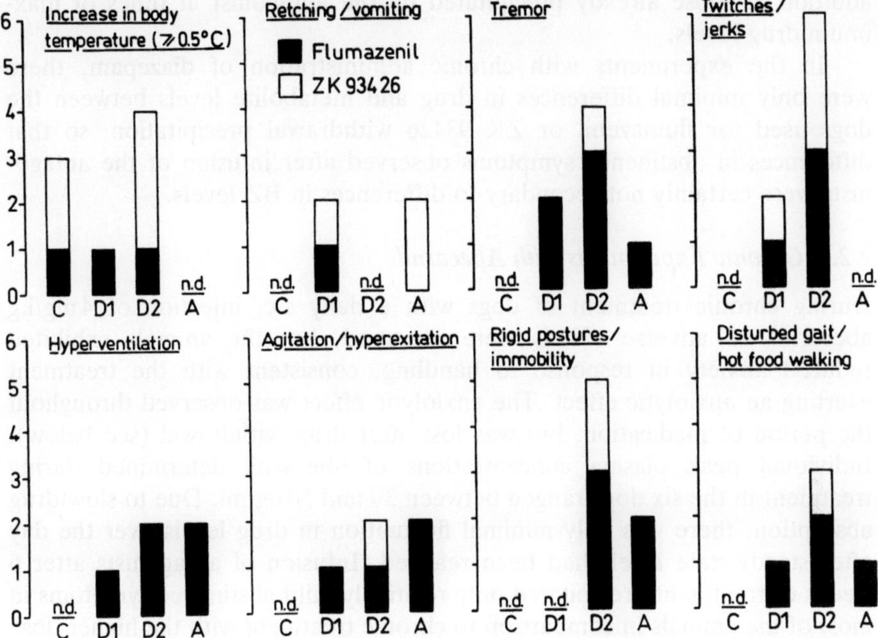

Fig. 2. Withdrawal signs precipitated by infusion of BZ-receptor antagonists after chronic treatment of six dogs with diazepam or abecarnil. Flumazenil and ZK 93426 were solubilized in 50% glycofurol in water at a concentration of 10 mg/ml and were infused i.v. at a rate of 3 ml/min up to a total dose of 20 mg/kg. Infusion of the antagonists was undertaken either in drug-naive dogs (*C*) or after chronic treatment of dogs with diazepam (1 h after the last oral dosing) or abecarnil (2 h after the last s.c. injection). Diazepam was either administered three times daily at 1 mg/kg po for 1 week (*D1*) or three times daily at 2 mg/kg po for 2 weeks (*D2*). Abecarnil (*A*) was administered once daily at 4 mg/kg s.c. for 6 weeks. The same dogs were used for all experiments with intervals of 3 months between each drug experiment. Three dogs of each experiment received flumazenil and the other three dogs received ZK 93426. The *bars* indicate the number of dogs displaying withdrawal signs during or after infusion of antagonist. Behavioral signs, i.e., ataxia, sedation, and vocalization (groaning, growling), induced by the antagonists in both drug-naive dogs and diazepam- or abecarnil-pretreated dogs are not shown; *n.d.* indicates "not determined", i.e. that the respective behavioural alteration was not observed

walking with tentative placement and rapid lifting of paws was observed in one animal), but showed twitches (one dog) or marked generalized myoclonic jerks (two dogs) during forward locomotion, which resembled the typical generalized epileptic myoclonic jerks of head or body which can be induced by PTZ in diazepam-naive dogs (Löscher 1983). Three hours after infusion, one dog exhibited a generalized tonic–clonic seizure, while another dog still showed myoclonic jerks. On the days after the last day of diazepam treatment, all six dogs behaved normally and showed no alterations in body weight or body temperature, indicating that the decline in diazepam and metabolite levels did not cause withdrawal symptoms in addition to those already precipitated by the antagonist at times of maximum drug levels.

In the experiments with chronic administration of diazepam, there were only minimal differences in drug and metabolite levels between the dogs used for flumazenil or ZK 93426 withdrawal precipitation, so that differences in abstinence symptoms observed after infusion of the antagonists were certainly not secondary to differences in BZ levels.

2.2.3 Chronic Experiments with Abecarnil

During chronic treatment of dogs with a daily s.c. injection of 4 mg/kg abecarnil no adverse effects were observed, but the animals exhibited reduced anxiety in response to handling, consistent with the treatment exerting an anxiolytic effect. The anxiolytic effect was observed throughout the period of medication, but was lost after drug withdrawal (see below). Individual peak plasma concentrations of abecarnil determined during treatment in the six dogs ranged between 30 and 50 ng/ml. Due to slow drug absorption, there was only minimal fluctuation in drug levels over the day after steady-state levels had been reached. Infusion of antagonists after 6 weeks of treatment precipitated only relatively mild abstinence symptoms in most of the animals in comparison to chronic treatment with the higher dose of diazepam (Fig. 2).

With flumazenil, two dogs became immobile: one of the animals stood motionless in a rigid posture for several minutes and was not able to move, the other animal exhibited a prone position (sternal recumbency) for about 15 min. The third dog showed a disturbed gait with retarded setting of forepaws, and transient tremor and circling. Two animals appeared hyperexcited shortly after infusion of flumazenil and showed transitory hyperventilation. With ZK 93426, the only withdrawal symptom observed was retching or vomiting in two of the dogs; otherwise the three animals behaved normally. In contrast to treatment with diazepam, none of the six animals chronically treated with abecarnil showed twitches, jerks, or seizures in response to the infusion of antagonists. Body temperature was not altered in any of the dogs. On the days after the last administration of abecarnil, no further behavioral alterations and no changes in body temperature or body weight were noted. However, the anxiolytic effect observed during treatment with abecarnil disappeared and the animals behaved as anxiously as prior to onset of chronic treatment.

2.2.4 Comparison of Withdrawal Signs After Diazepam and Abecarnil

When all individual withdrawal signs observed after injection of flumazenil or ZK 93426 were summed, the sum of signs in abecarnil-pretreated dogs was significantly lower than that of dogs treated with 6 mg/kg diazepam per day, but similar to that of dogs treated with 3 mg/kg diazepam per day (Fig. 3).

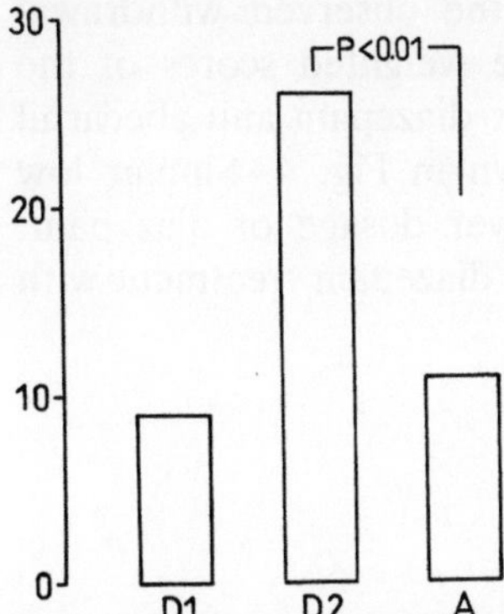

Fig. 3. Sum of individual withdrawal signs observed during or after i.v. infusion of flumazenil and ZK 93426 in six dogs treated with diazepam (*D1*, three times daily 1 mg/kg po for 1 week; *D2*, three times daily 2 mg/kg po for 2 weeks) or abecarnil (*A*, once daily 4 mg/kg s.c. for 6 weeks)

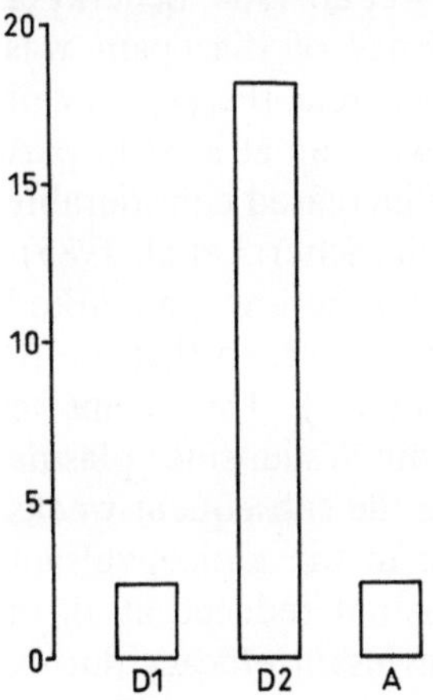

Fig. 4. Weighted scores received by using the Diazepam Withdrawal Scale (McNicholas et al. 1983) for withdrawal signs observed during or after i.v. infusion of flumazenil and ZK 93426 in six dogs treated with diazepam (*D1*, three times daily 1 mg/kg po for 1 week; *D2*, three times daily 2 mg/kg po for 2 weeks) or abecarnil (*A*, once daily 4 mg/kg s.c. for 6 weeks)

In addition to summing all behavioral alterations of diazepam- or abecarnil-pretreated dogs in response to BZ-receptor antagonists, the signs of withdrawal were weighted according to the "Diazepam Withdrawal Abstinence Scale" generated by McNicholas et al. (1983) for comparing withdrawal syndromes after chronic treatment with different BZ-receptor agonists. Weighting factors of this scale are 1 for gross tremor, 10 for tonic–clonic seizures and 1.4 for disturbed gait, such as stiff-legged walking.

Withdrawal scores were obtained by weighting the observed withdrawal signs by these factors and then summing up the weighted scores of the respective group of dogs (separately calculated for diazepam and abecarnil treatment). Data calculated in this way are shown in Fig. 4. Similar low scores were calculated for abecarnil and the lower dosage of diazepam, whereas markedly higher scores were obtained for diazepam treatment with 6 mg/kg per day (Fig. 4).

3 Discussion

The major finding of the experiments in dogs is that in contrast to BZ, chronic treatment with the BZ-receptor ligand, abecarnil, does not seem to induce marked tolerance and/or physical dependence. Indeed, previous experiments with diazepam and clonazepam in dogs, using a similar study protocol as in the present investigation, have shown a marked reduction in anticonvulsant efficacy during chronic treatment (Frey et al. 1984; Scherkl et al. 1985). As shown in Fig. 5, anticonvulsant efficacy of diazepam was almost totally lost after 1 week of daily treatment, whereas the potency of clonazepam declined more slowly, which, however, was due at least in part to the fact that plasma concentrations of clonazepam increased considerably in several dogs during the course of chronic medication (Scherkl et al. 1985). In contrast to diazepam and clonazepam, with abecarnil there was a marked increase in anticonvulsant efficacy after 1 week of treatment, so that the β-carboline reached the acute potency of diazepam (Fig. 5). This seems to suggest that accumulation of abecarnil occurred in brain tissue, since plasma levels did not explain the increase in efficacy. During the subsequent weeks of treatment with abecarnil, only a slight reduction in the anticonvulsant efficacy of the β-carboline took place or efficacy was not reduced at all in most dogs. Interestingly, a similar pattern of anticonvulsant efficacy during chronic treatment of dogs was recently reported for clorazepate (Fig. 5), a prodrug of desmethyldiazepam (Scherkl et al. 1989). Indeed, studies on binding characteristics and intrinsic activity have suggested that like abecarnil desmethyldiazepam behaves as a partial agonist at BZ receptors (Frey and Löscher 1982; Gobbi et al. 1987). However, in contrast to the present experiments with abecarnil, marked withdrawal symptoms, including seizures, were observed after cessation of treatment with clorazepate in dogs (Scherkl et al. 1989), confirming previous studies in dogs with chronic administration of desmethyldiazepam (McNicholas et al. 1985). This might indicate that the lack of tolerance and dependence during chronic treatment with abecarnil is not simply explained by partial agonism at BZ receptors. Indeed from behavioral experiments with abecarnil in rodents, it was suggested that abecarnil acts as a full agonist at subtype(s) of BZ receptors whose activation may account for the anxiolytic and anticonvulsant effects of

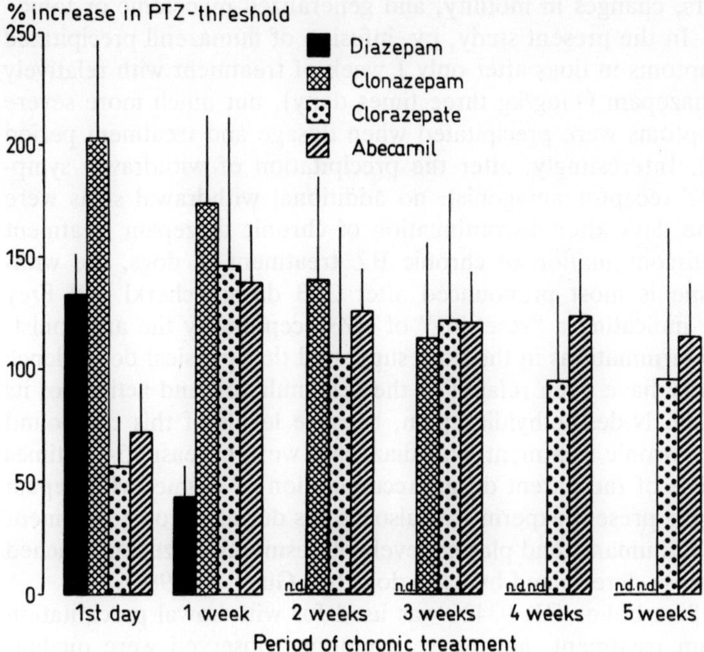

Fig. 5. Comparison of anticonvulsant potencies of diazepam, clonazepam, clorazepate, and abecarnil during chronic treatment in dogs. Data for diazepam and clonazepam were calculated from results of previous experiments with these drugs (Frey et al. 1984; Scherkl et al. 1985, 1989). Based on pharmacokinetic studies, diazepam was administered at 0.5 mg/kg po three times daily, clonazepam at 0.5 mg/kg po twice daily, clorazepate at 2 mg/kg po three times daily, and abecarnil at 4 mg/kg s.c. once daily. Before onset of chronic treatment and at weekly intervals during chronic treatment, the PTZ seizure threshold was determined 10 min after i.v. injection of 0.5 mg/kg diazepam, 0.1 mg/kg clonazepam, 2 mg/kg clorazepate, or 0.5 mg/kg abecarnil, respectively. For the calculation of percentage increases in the PTZ threshold after drug administration, PTZ thresholds determined in each dog 1 week before the first i.v. injection of BZ or abecarnil were used as control. Data are given as means ± SE of 3–9 dogs per experiment. *n.d.*, not determined. (From Löscher et al. 1990)

abecarnil, but as an antagonist or partial agonist at other receptor subtypes which may be important in the plethora of BZ functions (Stephens et al. 1990; Turski et al. 1990). Thus, abecarnil might be considered a subtype-specific BZ ligand rather than a partial agonist.

It has been demonstrated previously that abstinence symptoms can be precipitated by BZ-receptor antagonists after prolonged administration of BZs in monkeys, dogs, cats, or rodents (Cumin et al. 1982; McNicholas et al. 1983; Lukas and Griffiths 1984; Scherkl and Frey 1986; Giorgi et al. 1988; Wilson and Gallager 1988; Löscher et al. 1989). Withdrawal symptoms precipitated by BZ-receptor antagonists in these species included retching and vomiting, rigidity, decreased food intake, increased body temperature, anxiety, tremors, changes in motility, and generalized myoclonic or tonic–clonic seizures. In the present study, i.v. infusion of flumazenil precipitated abstinence symptoms in dogs after only 1 week of treatment with relatively low doses of diazepam (1 mg/kg three times daily), but much more severe abstinence symptoms were precipitated when dosage and treatment period were increased. Interestingly, after the precipitation of withdrawal symptoms by the BZ-receptor antagonist, no additional withdrawal signs were observed on the days after discontinuation of chronic diazepam treatment (after abrupt discontinuation of chronic BZ treatment in dogs, the withdrawal syndrome is most pronounced after 2–3 days; Scherkl and Frey 1986), possibly indicating a "resetting" of BZ receptors by the antagonist. Plasma level determinations in the dogs suggested that physical dependence on diazepam may have been related to the accumulation and actions of its major metabolite, N-desmethyldiazepam, because levels of this compound reached during chronic treatment with diazepam were at least 15–20 times higher than those of the parent drug. Accumulation of desmethyldiazepam as observed in the present experiments also occurs during chronic treatment with diazepam in humans, and plasma levels of desmethyldiazepam reached are similar to those determined by us in dogs (cf. Guentert 1984).

When the β-carboline ZK 93426 was used for withdrawal precipitation during diazepam treatment, abstinence symptoms observed were qualitatively and quantitatively different from those precipitated by flumazenil, thus substantiating previous experiments with both BZ-receptor antagonists in a larger group of diazepam-dependent dogs (Löscher et al. 1989). ZK 93426 is a BZ-receptor antagonist with a similar in vitro and in vivo potency as flumazenil (Jensen et al. 1984). In contrast to flumazenil, which exhibits slight partial agonistic and/or inverse agonistic activity at high doses (Corda et al. 1982; File et al. 1982; Haefely 1985), ZK 93426 is an almost neutral BZ-receptor ligand in most paradigms (Jensen et al. 1984; Löscher et al. 1985; De Deyn and Macdonald 1987). This is also demonstrated by the present experiments in diazepam-naive dogs, in which flumazenil induced sedation and marked ataxia in high doses, whereas ZK 93426 was devoid of typical BZ receptor-related effects.

Interesting differences in the precipitated withdrawal were found after prolonged treatment with diazepam and after the β-carboline abecarnil. The most marked (and possibly also most important) difference was that flumazenil and ZK 93426 produced severe (pro)convulsant effects in diazepam-pretreated dogs, whereas no such withdrawal signs were observed in dogs after chronic treatment with abecarnil. Indeed, by challenge with ZK 93426, the only abstinence effects observed in abecarnil-treated dogs were retching and vomiting.

Although abstinence symptoms precipitated in abecarnil-treated dogs were only mild, the presence of such abstinence symptoms indicated that some physical dependence had developed in most animals. In this respect it is interesting to note that previous experiments with diazepam in baboons have suggested that a history of BZ exposure sensitizes animals to a subsequent development of physical dependence (Lukas and Griffiths 1984). Thus, the fact that all dogs treated with abecarnil in this series of experiments had a history of chronic diazepam exposure might be important for the present results. Indeed, the initial study on chronic abecarnil in dogs (Fig. 1), in which no abstinence symptoms were observed upon discontinuation of treatment, was carried out in BZ-naive animals.

One might object that concentrations reached by the daily s.c. administration of 4 mg/kg abecarnil as suspension in peanut oil were too low to induce tolerance and dependence during chronic treatment. In this respect, it should be noted that at least three observations strongly indicate that pharmacologically relevant concentrations were reached by the s.c. administration of abecarnil: (1) during efficacy testing in the first chronic experiment with abecarnil, the anticonvulsant potency of i.v. injected abecarnil was markedly increased after 1 week of chronic s.c. treatment, thus indicating that the s.c. drug administration contributed significantly to the anticonvulsant activity determined after i.v. drug administration, (2) the PTZ threshold was still significantly increased 3 days after cessation of chronic s.c. administration, and (3) the plasma levels of abecarnil attained in dogs (10–50 ng/ml) in the two chronic experiments with 4 mg/kg per day were well above the plasma levels reached during treatment with effective doses (about 3–15 mg per day) of abecarnil in humans (Duka et al. 1989; Ballenger et al. 1991). In this respect, it is important to note that abecarnil has been shown to be two to ten times more potent than diazepam, e.g., in tests for anticonvulsant or anxiolytic activity (Stephens et al. 1990; Turski et al. 1990). Indeed, abecarnil's affinity for central BZ receptors is about 70 times higher than that of diazepam (Stephens et al. 1990). Thus, although plasma levels of abecarnil during chronic treatment of dogs at the s.c. dosage used in the present study were about 50–70 times lower than those of diazepam and its metabolites determined during treatment with 6 mg/kg per day diazepam, it can be assumed that both treatments resulted in a comparable BZ receptor occupancy (the distribution of abecarnil and diazepam and its metabolites in dogs is similar; Löscher and Frey 1981; Löscher et al. 1990). Furthermore, with respect to the differences in precipitated withdrawal between treatment with 4 mg/kg per day abecarnil and 6 mg/kg per day diazepam, one should consider that the duration of treatment with abecarnil was considerably longer (6 weeks) compared to diazepam (2 weeks). It has previously been shown in dogs that the severity of withdrawal signs is a function of dosage and duration of treatment (Löscher et al. 1989; Scherkl et al. 1985, 1989), so that the longer duration of treatment with abecarnil compared to diazepam would favor the development of physical dependence.

In conclusion, the present chronic dog experiments with abecarnil strongly indicate that this novel anxiolytic and anticonvulsant compound might have important advantages compared to traditional BZ-receptor agonists, such as diazepam, regarding both the induction of tolerance and of physical dependence. Phase I safety studies with single- and multiple-dose administration of abecarnil by the oral route have shown that abecarnil is well tolerated by humans, and that bioavailability is high enough for chronic anxiolytic or antiepileptic therapy by the oral route (Duka et al. 1989; Krause et al. 1990). Recent results from clinical studies in generalized anxiety disorder patients have shown abecarnil to be well tolerated and to be effective in alleviating anxiety symptoms in doses between 3 and 15 mg daily; moreover, no withdrawal symptoms occurred after acute discontinuation (Ballenger et al. 1991).

References

Ballenger JC, Mcdonald S, Noyes R, Rickels K, Sussman N, Woods S, Patin J, Singer J (1991) The first double-blind, placebo-controlled trial of a partial benzodiazepine agonist, abecarnil (ZK-112-119), in generalized anxiety disorder. Psychopharmacol Bull 27:171–179

Corda MG, Costa E, Guidotti A (1982) Specific proconvulsant action of an imidazobenzodiazepine (Ro 15-1788) on isoniazid convulsions. Neuropharmacology 21:91–94

Cumin R, Benetti EP, Scherschlicht R, Haefely WE (1982) Use of the specific benzodiazepine antagonist, Ro-15-1788, in studies of physiological dependence on benzodiazepines. Experentia 38:833–834

De Deyn PP, Macdonald RL (1987) CGS 9896 and ZK 91296, but not CGS 8216 and Ro 15-1788, are pure benzodiazepine antagonists on mouse neurons in culture. J Pharmacol Exp Ther 242:48–55

Duka T, Schütt B, Dorow R, McDonald S, Krause W, Fichte K (1989) ZK 112119, a β-carboline anxiolytic: phase I single- and multiple-dose studies to establish safety, tolerability and drug effects. Eur J Clin Pharmacol 36 [Suppl]:A48

File SE, Lister RG, Nutt DJ (1982) The anxiogenic action of benzodiazepine antagonists. Neuropharmacology 21:1033–1037

Frey H-H, Löscher W (1982) Anticonvulsant potency of unmetabolized diazepam. Pharmacology 25:154–159

Frey H-H, Philippin H-P, Scheuler W (1984) Development of tolerance to the anticonvulsant effect of diazepam in dogs. Eur J Pharmacol 104:27–38

Giorgi O, Corda MG, Fernandez A, Biggio G (1988) The abstinence syndrome in diazepam-dependent cats is precipitated by Ro 15-1788 and Ro 15-4513 but not by the benzodiazepine-receptor antagonist ZK 93426. Neurosci Lett 88:206–210

Gobbi M, Barone D, Mennini T, Garattini S (1987) Diazepam and desmethyldiazepam differ in their affinities and efficacies at "central" and "peripheral" benzodiazepine receptors. J Pharm Pharmacol 39:388–391

Guentert TW (1984) Pharmacokinetics of benzodiazepines and their metabolites. In: Bridges JW, Chasseaud LF (eds) Progress in drug etabolism, vol 8. Tayler and Francis, London, pp 241–386

Haefely W (1985) Pharmacology of benzodiazepine antagonists. Pharmacopsychiatry 18:163–166

Haefely W, Martin JR, Schoch P (1990) Novel anxiolytics that act as partial agonists at benzodiazepine receptors. Trends Pharmacol Sci 11:452–456

Haigh JRM, Feely M (1988) Tolerance to the anticonvulsant effect of benzodiazepines. Trends Pharmacol Sci 9:361–391

Jensen LH, Petersen EN, Braestrup C, Honoré T, Kehr W, Stephens DN, Schneider H, Seidelmann D, Schmiechen R (1984) Evaluation of the β-carboline ZK 93426 as a benzodiazepine-receptor antagonist. Psychopharmacology 83:249–256

Krause W, Mengel H, Nordholm L (1989) Determination of β-carboline derivatives in biological samples by high-performance liquid chromatography with fluorescence detection. J Pharm Sci 78:622–626

Krause W, Schütt B, Duka T (1990) Pharmacokinetics and acute toleration of the β-carboline derivative abecarnil in man. Arzneimittelforschung (Drug Res) 40:529–532

Löscher W (1982) Relationship between GABA concentrations in cerebrospinal fluid and seizure excitability. J Neurochem 38:293–295

Löscher W (1983) Alterations in CSF GABA levels and seizure susceptibility developing during repeated administration of pentetrazole in dogs. Effects of acetylenic GABA, valproic acid and phenobarbital. Neurochem Int 5:405–412

Löscher W, Frey H-H (1981) Pharmacokinetics of diazepam in the dog. Arch Int Pharmacodyn Ther 254:180–196

Löscher W, Rundfeldt C (1990) Development of tolerance to clobazam in fully kindled rats: effects of intermittent flumazenil administration. Eur J Pharmacol 180:255–271

Löscher W, Schneider H, Kehr W (1985) Evaluation of different β-carbolines in Mongolian gerbils with reflex epilepsy. Eur J Pharmacol 114:261–266

Löscher W, Hönack D, Hashem A (1987) Anticonvulsant efficacy of clonazepam and the β-carboline ZK 93423 during chronic treatment in amygdala-kindled rats. Eur J Pharmacol 143:403–414

Löscher W, Hönack D, Faßbender CP (1989) Physical dependence on diazepam in the dog: precipitation of different abstinence syndromes by the benzodiazepine-receptor antagonists Ro 15–1788 and ZK 93426. Br J Pharmacol 97:843–852

Löscher W, Hönack D, Scherkl R, Hashem A, Frey H-H (1990) Pharmacokinetics, anticonvulsant efficacy and adverse effects of the β-carboline abecarnil, a novel ligand for benzodiazepine receptors, after acute and chronic administration in dogs. J Pharmacol Exp Ther 255:541–548

Löscher W, Rundfeldt D, Hönack D (1991) Tolerance to anticonvulsant effects of the partial benzodiazepine-receptor agonist abecarnil in kindled rats involves learning. Eur J Pharmacol 202:303–310

Lukas SE, Griffiths RR (1984) Precipitated diazepam withdrawal in baboons: effect of dose and duration of diazepam exposure. Eur J Pharmacol 100:163–171

McNicholas LF, Martin WR, Cherian S (1983) Physical dependence on diazepam and lorazepam in the dog. J Pharmacol Exp Ther 226:783–789

Owen RT, Tyrer (1983) Benzodiazepine dependence: a review of the evidence. Drugs 25:385–398

Scherkl R, Frey H-H (1986) Physical dependence on clonazepam in dogs. Pharmacology 32:18–24

Scherkl R, Scheuler W, Frey H-H (1985) Anticonvulsant effect of clonazepam in the dog: development of tolerance and physical dependence. Arch Int Pharmacodyn Ther 278:249–260

Scherkl R, Kurudi D, Frey H-H (1989) Clorazepate in dogs: tolerance to the anticonvulsant effect and signs of physical dependence. Epilepsy Res 3:144–150

Schneider HH, Turski L, Krause W, Stephens DN (1990) Short- and long-term tolerance to abecarnil, a beta-carboline benzodiazepine-receptor ligand: antagonism of PTZ convulsion threshold vs. receptor occupation and plasma level in the mouse. Soc Neurosci Abstr 16:1037

Stephens DN, Schneider HH, Kehr W, Andrews JS, Retting K-J, Turski L, Schmiechen R, Turner JD, Jensen LH, Petersen EN, Honoré T, Bondo Hansen J (1990) Abecarnil, a metabolically stable, anxioselective β-carboline acting at benzodiazepine receptors. J Pharmacol Exp Ther 253:334–343

Stephens DN, Schneider HH, Turski L, Hillmann M, Huba R, Turner JD (1991) Abecarnil: A β-carboline anxiolytic showing a selective action at central benzodiazepine receptors. Soc Neurosci Abstr 17:1342

Turski L, Stephens DN, Jensen LH, Petersen EN, Meldrum BS, Patel S, Bondo Hansen J, Löscher W, Schneider HH, Schmiechen R (1990) Anticonvulsant action of the β-carboline abecarnil – Studies in rodents and baboon, Papio papio. J Pharmacol Exp Ther 253:344–352

Wilson MA, Gallager DW (1988) Ro 15-1788-induced seizures in rats continually exposed to diazepam for prolonged periods. Epilepsy Res 2:14–19
Wilson JI, Feely M, Gent JP (1989) Apparent separation of benzodiazepine tolerance and dependence: flumazenil does not abolish the withdrawal effect. Br J Pharmacol 96:676P
Woods JH, Katz JL, Winger G (1987) Abuse liability of benzodiazepines. Pharmacol Rev 39:251–419

Behavioral Pharmacology of Abecarnil in Baboons: Reduced Dependence and Abuse Potential

C.A. Sannerud[1,3], N.A. Ator[1], and R.R. Griffiths[1,2]

1 Introduction

Abecarnil (isopropyl 6-benzyloxy-4-methoxymethyl-β-carboline-3-carboxylate; ZK 112,119), which is a β-carboline, exerts pharmacological effects at the benzodiazepine binding site on the gamma-aminobutyric acid type A (GABA$_A$)-receptor complex. Its distinct profile of biochemical and behavioral effects has been suggested to indicate partial and/or selective benzodiazepine-receptor activity (Stephens et al. 1990). A series of experiments in baboons further characterized the behavioral pharmacological profile of abecarnil and provides information about its relative abuse liability (Sannerud et al. 1992). Specifically, tolerance, withdrawal, self-injection, and drug discrimination were evaluated with abecarnil using methods for which data have been previously reported for benzodiazepines and related novel compounds.

2 Chronic Abecarnil Administration

Four benzodiazepine-naive baboons were surgically prepared with chronically indwelling i.g. catheters to study the effects of abecarnil and its withdrawal (cf. Sannerud et al. 1992). Baboons were trained to respond under a fixed-ratio (FR) 30 schedule of reinforcement. During a 2-week baseline phase, suspending agent vehicle was administered through the i.g. catheter during 24 h. During the 6- to 8-week chronic administration phase, baboons received 100 mg/kg abecarnil per day via continuous i.g. infusion. In order to assess precipitated withdrawal from abecarnil, an injection of flumazenil (Ro 15-1788, 5.0 mg/kg, i.m.) was given to each baboon on day 8 of chronic

[1] Department of Psychiatry and Behavioral Sciences, The Johns Hopkins University School of Medicine, Baltimore, MD 21205, USA
[2] Department of Neuroscience, The John Hopkins University School of Medicine, Baltimore, MD 21205, USA
[3] Behavioral Pharmacology and Genetics Laboratory, NIDA–Addiction Research Center, Baltimore, MD 21224, USA

administration. During the 4-week spontaneous withdrawal phase, vehicle alone was substituted for abecarnil.

2.1 Behavioral Observations

In addition to recording daily food-pellet intake during this study, 1-h observational sessions were conducted systematically prior to, during, and after chronic abecarnil administration using the behavioral rating scale described by Sannerud et al. (1991).

Chronic administration of 100 mg/kg abecarnil per day produced few behavioral signs of sedation in the four baboons (Sannerud et al. 1992). During the first week of chronic abecarnil administration, two baboons showed intention tremor (indicative of ataxia) and one baboon displayed lip droop. In contrast, acute administration of high doses of benzodiazepines to baboons produced behavioral signs of ataxia, incoordination, and sedation (Lukas and Griffiths 1982; Lamb and Griffiths 1984; Sannerud et al. 1989, 1991). The data from the present study are consistent with reports that

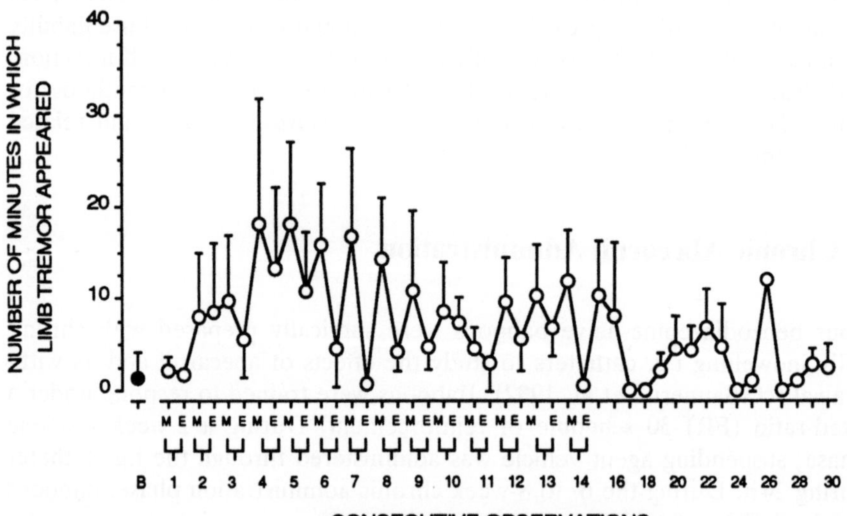

Fig. 1. Group mean frequency of limb tremor in baboons before and after chronic 100 mg/kg per day abecarnil administration ($n = 4$). *Y-axis*, the number of minutes during the 60-min observational session in which limb tremor occurred. The vehicle substitution phase was conducted for 4 weeks; observational sessions were performed twice daily for the first 2 weeks (*M*, morning; *E*, evening), then approximately two or three times weekly for the duration of this phase. *Numerals* indicate consecutive days of vehicle substitution; *closed symbol* above *B*, the grand mean score in five observational sessions during the 2-week baseline period prior to the start of chronic abecarnil administration; *open symbols*, mean score during vehicle substitution; *brackets*, ±1 SE; *absence of bracket*, SE less than the diameter of the symbol

abecarnil has a weak muscle-relaxant effect when compared to diazepam (Stephens et al. 1990; Löscher et al. 1990).

The present study found that chronic high-dose abecarnil administration produced mild physical dependence, evidenced by the low frequency of withdrawal signs after either flumazenil administration or vehicle substitution. Flumazenil given on day 8 of chronic abecarnil administration produced vomiting in one baboon, increases in limb tremor in three baboons, and increases in muscle twitch/jerk in two baboons compared to the previous 7 days of chronic abecarnil administration, and compared to the effects of flumazenil in drug-free baboons (Sannerud et al. 1992). Spontaneous withdrawal from abecarnil (vehicle substitution) produced transitory increases in some mild signs of benzodiazepine withdrawal, such as limb tremor (Fig. 1), body tremor, scratching, and abnormal postures in some baboons. These mild withdrawal signs increased over predrug levels on days 2–5 after termination of abecarnil, and tended to decrease toward predrug levels during the 30-day withdrawal period (Sannerud et al. 1992).

2.2 Food Intake

Figure 2 shows mean food-pellet intake before and during chronic abecarnil administration, and during 4 weeks of vehicle substitution. Although food-pellet intake was variable within and across baboons, abecarnil administration appeared to increase food-pellet intake. Vehicle substitution after

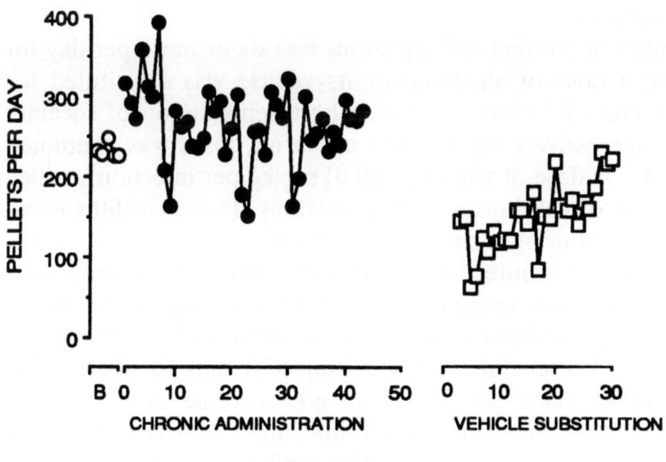

Fig. 2. Group mean food-pellet intake in baboons before, during, and after chronic administration of 100 mg/kg abecarnil ($n = 4$). Data points in each panel show food-pellet intake during predrug vehicle baseline (*B, open squares*), 6 weeks of 6- to 8-week chronic 100 mg/kg per day abecarnil administration (*filled circles*), and 4 weeks of vehicle substitution (*open circles*)

chronic abecarnil administration was associated with a decrease in the number of pellets, which subsequently increased toward vehicle control levels.

The profile of behavioral signs and changes in food intake observed under conditions of precipitated and spontaneous withdrawal from abecarnil suggested mild benzodiazepine-like withdrawal symptoms (cf. Griffiths and Sannerud 1987). However, in previous research with chronic benzodiazepines, there was a higher incidence (100%) of the more severe precipitated withdrawal sign of vomiting after 7 days of administration of diazepam (Lukas and Griffiths 1982) and lorazepam (Lamb and Griffiths 1984) than after 8 days of abecarnil (25%) in the present study. This difference is consistent with a recent report in dogs indicating a less severe spontaneous and precipitated withdrawal syndrome after abecarnil than after classic benzodiazepines (Löscher et al. 1990).

3 Self-Injection

Baboons, surgically prepared with chronically indwelling i.v. silastic catheters, were trained to self-inject cocaine (0.32 mg/kg per injection) under a cocaine-substitution procedure described elsewhere (Griffiths et al. 1992). Drug injections were available under an FR 80 or 160 response schedule on the drug lever. A 3-h timeout period limited the number of injections to eight a day. Food pellets were available 24 h a day under an FR 30 response schedule on a second lever.

When the number of cocaine self-injections was six or more per day for 3 consecutive days, a dose of abecarnil or its vehicle was substituted for cocaine for a minimum of 15 days, followed by a reinstitution of cocaine. This procedure of successively substituting abecarnil doses was continued throughout the study. A dose of triazolam (0.01 mg/kg per injection), which maintained peak rates of self-injection in a previous study (Griffiths et al. 1991), was also evaluated using identical procedures.

Response-contingent i.v. injections of abecarnil maintained mean rates of responding similar to those maintained by response-contingent i.v. injections of abecarnil vehicle, and lower than those maintained by both cocaine and triazolam. Figure 3 presents the mean self-injection data for abecarnil in three baboons. The standard dose of 0.32 mg/kg cocaine and 0.1 mg/kg triazolam maintained high daily rates of self-injection. Vehicle substitution resulted in low levels of self-injection. Abecarnil (0.032–1.0 mg/kg per injection) maintained mean rates of self-injection that were generally similar to vehicle. The highest dose of abecarnil tested (1.0 mg/kg per injection) produced signs of sedation (ataxia, lip droop) in two of the three baboons, and decreased food-pellet intake in one baboon. These data indicate that over a wide range of doses abecarnil does not serve as an effective reinforcer

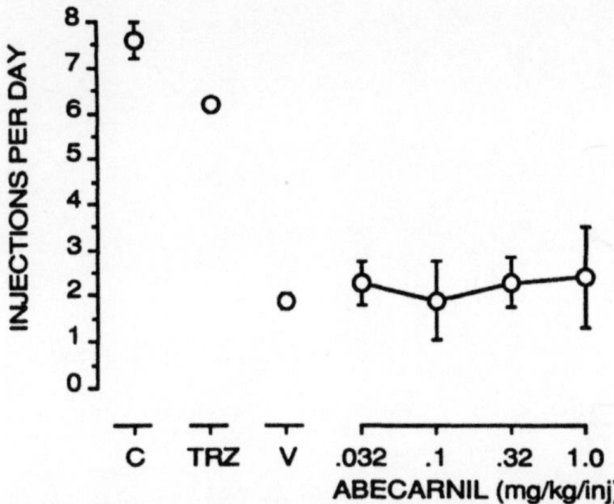

Fig. 3. Group mean number of injections per day in baboons of abecarnil, abecarnil vehicle (*V*), or triazolam (*TRZ*) (0.01 mg/kg) after substitution for cocaine (*C*; *n* = 3). Data point above *C* represents the grand mean for the 3 days of cocaine HCl (0.32 mg/kg per injection) availability that preceded each abecarnil dose or vehicle. Drug data points indicate grand mean of the last 5 days after substitution of an abecarnil dose, abecarnil vehicle, or 0.01 mg/kg triazolam substitution. *Brackets*, ±1 SE; *absence of bracket*, SE less than the diameter of the symbol

in the baboon under experimental conditions in which self-injection was maintained with a variety of other sedatives/anxiolytics (Griffiths et al. 1981, 1991).

Abecarnil's lack of reinforcing efficacy cannot be attributed to a lack of biological/behavioral activity of abecarnil in baboons or to a behavioral suppressant effect of the abecarnil vehicle itself. The highest dose of abecarnil produced sedation in two of the three baboons, and cocaine dissolved in abecarnil vehicle maintained high rates of self-injection (Sannerud et al. 1992).

4 Drug Discrimination Study

Four baboons were trained to discriminate lorazepam (1.8 mg/kg po, administered 60 min before the session) from the no-drug (i.e., no dosing) condition using a procedure described in more detail elsewhere (cf. Ator and Griffiths 1986). The discriminative–stimulus effects of abecarnil (0.32–32 mg/kg po) and its vehicle were evaluated at 1 h, and on some test days also at 3, 5, 7, 9, 11, 13, and 15 h after drug or placebo administration.

Results with abecarnil 1 h after administration were inconsistent within and across baboons. Abecarnil produced only 24% and 48% mean drug-lever responding after doses of 18 and/or 32 mg/kg po, respectively (Fig. 4). Individual data showed clear abecarnil generalization (i.e., >80% drug-appropriate responding in two determinations) occurred for only one of the

                                                        C.A. Sannerud et al.

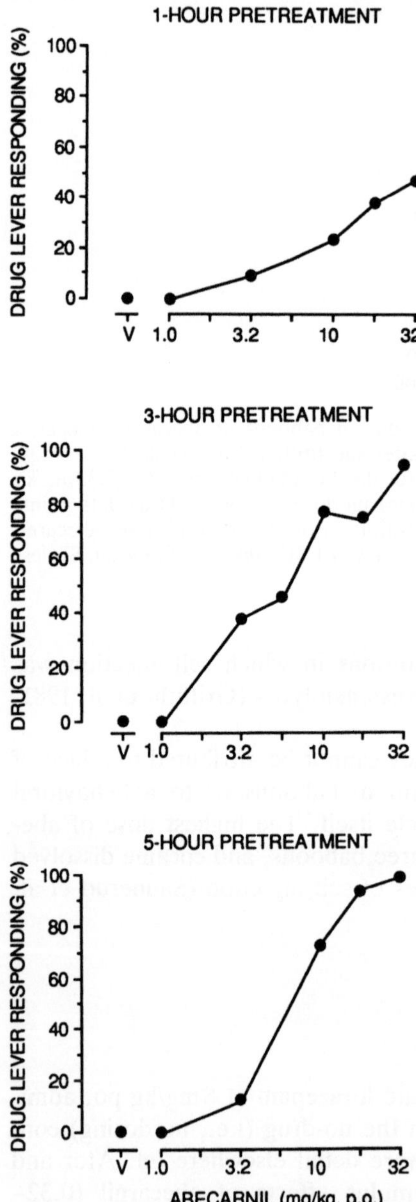

Fig. 4. Group mean percentages of total session responding on the drug lever in test sessions conducted 1, 3, and 5h after. The administration of abecarnil or the quinine placebo (V) po to baboons trained to discriminate lorazepam (1.8 mg/kg po) from the no-drug condition ($n = 4$)

four baboons. A time-course study of abecarnil showed a dose-dependent generalization to abecarnil, with maximal drug-lever responding occurring reliably in all baboons 3–5 h after 18–32 mg/kg abecarnil po (Fig. 4). The duration of drug-lever responding differed across baboons, but it generally decreased by 9–13 h after administration of the two highest doses. Response rates after any dose of abecarnil were generally not different from control at any time point after administration. The discriminative–stimulus effects of abecarnil were most likely mediated at the benzodiazepine receptor since flumazenil (0.32 mg/kg, i.m.) completely antagonized the abecarnil discriminative stimulus tested 5 h after abecarnil doses of 3.2, 10, 18, and 32 mg/kg.

Benzodiazepines and some nonbenzodiazepine ligands for the benzodiazepine receptor generally have produced dose-related increases in drug-lever responding in virtually all baboons trained to discriminate lorazepam when tested at a standard pretreatment time of 60 min (Ator and Griffiths 1986, 1989). The apparent delayed onset of discriminative–stimulus effects of abecarnil observed in the present study is noteworthy. Since abecarnil does not produce active metabolites (Krause and Mengel 1990; Krause et al. 1990), the delayed onset of its discriminative–stimulus effects in baboons may be due to slow absorption (cf. Krause et al. 1990).

5 Conclusion

The behavioral profile of abecarnil in the baboon was novel compared to classic benzodiazepine agonists. Although abecarnil produced discriminative–stimulus effects similar to classic benzodiazepines, it produced relatively less sedation, physical dependence, and drug reinforcement. The results of the present study are consistent with the suggestion that abecarnil, with its novel profile of behavioral and pharmacological effects, may be a partial and/or selective agonist at the $GABA_A$-receptor complex (Stephens et al. 1990). In addition, the failure of abecarnil to maintain i.v. self-administration and the delayed onset of discriminative–stimulus effects after oral administration suggest that this novel anxiolytic may have a reduced risk of abuse by drug abusers.

Acknowledgements. The data in this paper are based on that reported in Sannerud et al. (1992). Different portions of this research were supported by NIDA Contract 271-86-8113, NIDA grants RO1 DA01147 and RO1 DA04133, and a grant from Schering AG, Berlin, Germany.

References

Ator NA, Griffiths RR (1986) Discriminative–stimulus effects of atypical anxiolytics in baboons and rats. J Pharmacol Exp Ther 237:393–403

Ator NA, Griffiths RR (1989) Asymmetrical cross-generalization in drug discrimination with lorazepam and pentobarbital training conditions. Drug Dev Res 16:355–364

Griffiths RR, Lukas SE, Bradford LD, Brady JV, Snell JD (1981) Self-injection of barbiturates and benzodiazepines in the baboon. Psychopharmacology 75:101–109

Griffiths RR, Lamb RJ, Sannerud CA, Ator NA, Brady JV (1991) Self-injection of barbiturates, benzodiazepines and other sedative-anxiolytics in baboons. Psychopharmacology 103:154–161

Griffiths RR, Sannerud CA, Ator NA, Brady JV (1992) Zolpidem behavioral pharmacology in baboons: self-injection, discrimination, tolerance and withdrawal. J Pharmacol Exp Ther 260:1199–1208

Griffiths RR, Sannerud CA (1987) Abuse of and dependence on benzodiazepines and other anxiolytic/sedative drugs. In: Meltzer H (ed) Psychopharmacology, The Third Generation of Progress. Raven Press, New York, pp 1535–1541

Krause W, Mengel H (1990) Pharmacokinetics of the anxiolytic β-carboline derivative in the mouse, rat, rabbit, dog, cynomologous monkey, and baboon. Studies on species differences. Arzneimittelforschung (Drug Res) 40:522–529

Krause W, Schütt B, Duka T (1990) Pharmacokinetic and acute toleration of the β-carboline derivative abecarnil in man. Arzneimittelforschung (Drug Res) 40:529–532

Lamb RJ, Griffiths RR (1984) Precipitated and spontaneous withdrawal in baboons after chronic dosing with lorazepam and CGS 9896. Drug Alcohol Depend 14:11–17

Löscher W, Hönack D, Scherkl R, Hashem A, Frey HH (1990) Pharmacokinetics, anticonvulsant efficacy and adverse effects of the β-carboline abecarnil, a novel ligand for benzodiazepine receptors, after acute and chronic administration in dogs. J Pharmacol Exp Ther 255:541–548

Lukas SE, Griffiths RR (1982) Precipitated withdrawal by a benzodiazepine-receptor antagonist (Ro 15-1788) after 7 days of diazepam. Science 217:1161

Sannerud CA, Cook JM, Griffiths RR (1989) Behavioral differentiation of benzodiazepine ligands after repeated administration in baboons. Eur J Pharmacol 167:333–343

Sannerud CA, Allen M, Cook JM, Griffiths RR (1991) Behavioral effects of benzodiazepine ligands in non-dependent, diazepam-dependent and diazepam-withdrawn baboons. Eur J Pharmacol 202:159–169

Sannerud CA, Ator NA, Griffiths RR (1992) Behavioral pharmacology of abecarnil in baboons: self-injection, drug discrimination and physical dependence. Behav Pharmacol 3:507–516

Stephens DN, Schneider HH, Kehr W, Andrews JS, Rettig KJ, Turski L, Schmiechen R, Turner JD, Jensen LH, Petersen EN, Honoré T, Bondo Hansen J (1990) Abecarnil, a metabolically stable, anxioselective β-carboline acting at benzodiazepine receptors. J Pharmacol Exp Ther 253:334–343

Abecarnil Used to Treat Benzodiazepine Withdrawal

M.W. EMMETT-OGLESBY, D.A. LYTLE, and S.A. ENGLISH

1 Introduction

Dependence on sedative hypnotics encompasses a variety of drugs that share effects, in part or whole, when given acutely. Although the acute effects of these compounds may vary, from the standpoint of dependence, they all produce a characteristic set of signs (objectively verifiable events) and symptoms (subjectively perceived phenomena) upon termination of high-dose, long-term use. Indeed, the shared aspects of this withdrawal syndrome (Jaffe 1990) are the most compelling reason to link the drugs as a common group. Signs of sedative-hypnotic withdrawal can include such florid manifestations as grand mal convulsions; however, simply because symptoms do not have vivid manifestations, their role in the maintenance of chronic drug use should not be dismissed lightly. Among other considerations, symptoms of sedative-hypnotic withdrawal precede the onset of signs; these symptoms are aversive and the reinstatement of the drug of dependence terminates the symptoms. Thus, we have argued that the occurrence of anxiety, a key symptom of benzodiazepine withdrawal, may be critical in the maintenance of chronic benzodiazepine taking (Emmett-Oglesby et al. 1990).

Can abecarnil be used to treat benzodiazepine dependence? A positive answer to this question requires empirical evidence from two types of experiments. First, does abecarnil suppress signs and (particularly) symptoms of benzodiazepine withdrawal? Second, in subjects dependent on a benzodiazepine that are switched to abecarnil, does withdrawal occur when abecarnil is terminated? In addition to these two demonstrations, particularly because abecarnil is likely to be used chronically in patients suffering from anxiety, a third question must be answered: does abecarnil given chronically produce dependence/withdrawal? In this chapter, we will present evidence that abecarnil can be used to treat benzodiazepine withdrawal, and that when compared to benzodiazepines, the termination of chronic abecarnil appears to have many fewer withdrawal-producing effects.

Our evidence concerning abecarnil and dependence/withdrawal comes from drug-discrimination studies in animals (rats). Drug discrimination is

Department of Pharmacology, Texas College of Osteopathic Medicine, Fort Worth, TX 76107-2699, USA widely accepted as a model of human subjective drug effects (for an evaluation of the evidence regarding this proposition, see Preston and Bigelow 1991). In a drug-discrimination study, obtaining a reinforcer such as food is contingent upon emitting a correct response (for example, pressing only one of two available levers). The animal is trained to detect the stimulus effects of a drug by arbitrarily assigning one of the possible responses (e.g., presses on one of two levers) to the training-drug condition, and the other possible response to the vehicle condition. In practice, subjects are injected with drug or vehicle shortly before entering an operant chamber. When injected with drug, only responses on one of the levers will be reinforced with food; when injected with vehicle, only responses on the other lever will produce food. By this method, subjects come to discriminate the effects of the drug; when injected with a novel compound, they respond on the training-drug lever to the extent that the test compound produces effects that mimic those of the training drug.

In one of our models, rats were trained to discriminate the putative anxiogenic drug pentylenetetrazole (PTZ) from 0.9% saline. In this model, when subjects are treated with high doses of benzodiazepine agonists for several days, and are then treated with the benzodiazepine antagonist, flumazenil, to precipitate a state of withdrawal, they behave under flumazenil treatment as they had been trained to behave in response to PTZ. In drug-discrimination terminology, they substitute flumazenil for PTZ. Thus the internal stimulus provided in benzodiazepine-dependent rats by flumazenil-induced withdrawal, resembles that produced acutely by PTZ. (For an evaluation of the strengths and weaknesses of the PTZ discrimination in the assessment of anxiety-related aspects of benzodiazepine withdrawal see reviews by Lal and Emmett-Oglesby 1983; Emmett-Oglesby et al. 1990.) In the PTZ discrimination we determined the ability of (a) abecarnil to block the PTZ stimulus, (b) flumazenil to reverse this blocking action of abecarnil, (c) flumazenil or abecarnil to produce a PTZ-like stimulus following chronic administration of a benzodiazepine, and (d) flumazenil to precipitate a PTZ-like stimulus during chronic administration of abecarnil.

In a second model of benzodiazepine withdrawal, rats were maintained chronically on chlordiazepoxide (100 mg/kg per day) and trained to discriminate flumazenil from vehicle (3% carboxymethylcellulose). In this discrimination, precipitated withdrawal from benzodiazepine dependence appears to serve as the controlling stimulus (see review by Emmett-Oglesby and Rowan (1991) for an evaluation of the utility of this discrimination in the assessment of benzodiazepine withdrawal). In this discrimination we determined the ability of abecarnil to (a) substitute for flumazenil and (b) block spontaneous withdrawal from chlordiazepoxide. Based upon the time course for chlordiazepoxide withdrawal, we also determined whether abecarnil, given over this time course, would block the withdrawal-related stimulus, and then upon termination of abecarnil, whether a stimulus related to abecarnil withdrawal would occur.

2 Experiments Using PTZ Discrimination

Thirty male Long-Evans rats were trained to discriminate PTZ (17.8 mg/kg) from saline (0.9% solution) in conventional two-lever operant chambers (Coulbourn Instruments) using 45 mg food pellets (Bioserve) as a reinforcer. They were trained under a schedule of reinforcement in which ten responses (FR 10) were required to receive reinforcement.

The animals were injected with PTZ or saline, placed in the chamber 15 min later, and allowed to respond under the FR 10 schedule until 50 reinforcers were received or until 10 min had elapsed. For this training, responses on the correct lever (the PTZ lever following PTZ injection, or the saline lever following saline injection) were reinforced. Incorrect responses were counted but not reinforced. Selection of the correct lever was based on the criterion that at the start of the session, 10 responses resulting in reinforcement must be emitted on the injection-appropriate lever with fewer than 10 responses being emitted on the incorrect lever.

The criterion for discriminative control was defined as ten out of ten sessions in which correct lever selection occurred (at the start of the session, 10 responses were emitted on the injection-appropriate lever prior to 10 responses on the incorrect lever). Subsequently, animals were used for testing if they maintained a criterion of at least four out of five training sessions with correct lever selection.

For substitution tests, the test session was comparable to the training session, except that subjects were injected with the compound to be tested, and they were allowed to respond until only the first reinforcer was received, after which they were immediately removed from the chamber. For blocking tests, the test drug was injected shortly prior to the injection of either the training drug or the vehicle. Subjects were placed in the chamber 15 min after injection of the training drug, and the blocking test was then run identically to a substitution test.

The data were scored as the percent of subjects selecting the training-drug lever. If this percentage was 75% or greater, full substitution for the training stimulus is considered to have occurred. If this percentage was 25% or less, failure to substitute for the training stimulus is considered to have occurred. If subjects failed to complete 10 responses on one of the levers during the test session, they were not included in the calculation of percent of subjects selecting the drug lever.

In subjects trained to detect PTZ, either chlordiazepoxide or abecarnil fully blocked the PTZ stimulus in a dose-related manner (Fig. 1). Abecarnil was approximately ten times more potent than chlordiazepoxide in this regard (ED_{50}s by Litchfield-Wilcoxon analysis are 1.13 and 0.18 mg/kg for chlordiazepoxide and abecarnil, respectively). This PTZ-blocking effect of abecarnil was mediated by benzodiazepine receptors (Fig. 2), as shown by the ability of flumazenil to prevent the PTZ-blocking effect of abecarnil.

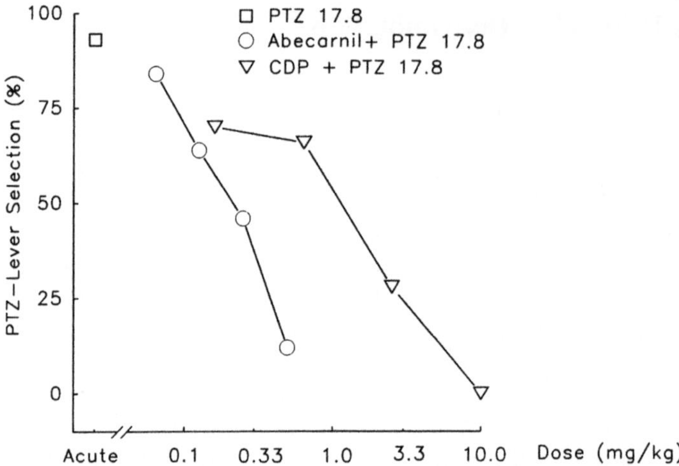

Fig. 1. Blocking effects of abecarnil and chlordiazepoxide (*CDP*) on the discriminative stimulus produced by pentylenetetrazole (*PTZ*). *Ordinate*, percent of subjects selecting the PTZ lever (a score of 0 equals all subjects selecting the vehicle lever). *Abscissa*, dose of either abecarnil or chlordiazepoxide. Rats trained to detect PTZ (17.8 mg/kg) versus vehicle (0.9% saline) were treated with either abecarnil or chlordiazepoxide, then 15 min later they received PTZ, and 15 min after PTZ they were tested for lever selection. *n* averages 12, and ranges from 8 to 15 for the various doses of abecarnil or chlordiazepoxide

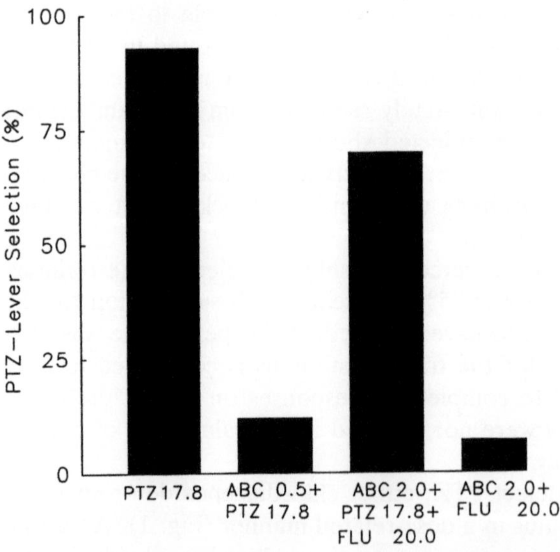

Fig. 2. Blockade of the pentylenetetrazole (*PTZ*) stimulus by abecarnil (*ABC*) and antagonism of this blockade by flumazenil (*FLU*). *Ordinate*, see Fig. 1. Subjects were tested with the treatment shown on the *abscissa*; numbers next to the drug symbols refer to dose, in mg/kg. PTZ was always given 15 min pretest, abecarnil was given 30 min pretest, and flumazenil was given 20 min pretest. The blockade of PTZ by abecarnil was antagonized by flumazenil and as shown in the *right-hand* column, this effect was not attributable to the combination of flumazenil and abecarnil producing a PTZ-like stimulus. *n* range from 8 to 16

The flumazenil reversal of abecarnil's blockade of the PTZ cue was not attributable to any direct PTZ-like effects of flumazenil, because when given by itself, flumazenil did not substitute for PTZ.

In contrast to the failure of flumazenil to substitute for PTZ when tested in nondependent subjects, following chronic chlordiazepoxide administration, 100 mg/kg per day for 7 days in two divided feedings via a nutritionally complete liquid diet, flumazenil substituted for PTZ (Fig. 3). Full substitution occurred 12 h after the last dose of chlordiazepoxide, and this substitution declined to vehicle-lever selection when flumazenil was tested over the next several days. Abecarnil produced a different pattern of results when tested in subjects that had received chlordiazepoxide chronically (Fig. 3), failing to substitute for chlordiazepoxide over the 6-day test period.

At doses of 1 or 2 mg/kg abecarnil is effective for at least 6 h in blocking the detection of PTZ (data not shown). Based upon these time-course data to determine whether abecarnil given chronically would produce dependence in the PTZ model, subjects were treated every 8 h with abecarnil (one group received 2 mg/kg and a second group received 4 mg/kg) for 6

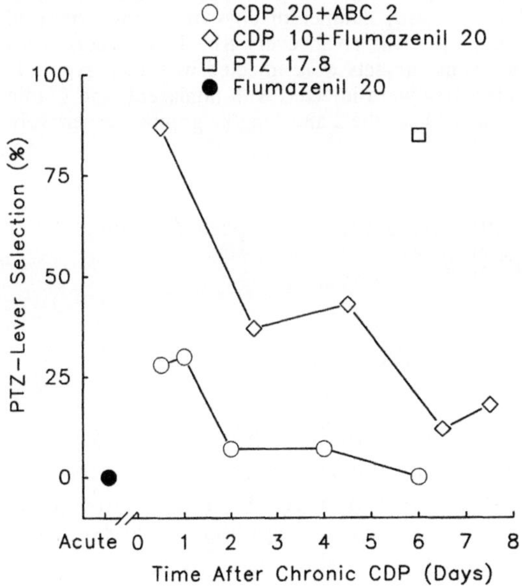

Fig. 3. Substitution of flumazenil, and failure of abecarnil (*ABC*) substitution, for pentylenetetrazole (*PTZ*) following chronic treatment with chlordiazepoxide (*CDP*). *Ordinate*, see Fig. 1. *Abscissa*, time since the termination of chronic chlordiazepoxide. Twelve hours following the last administration of chlordiazepoxide, subjects were tested with either flumazenil or abecarnil. For all of these tests, a small dose af chlordiazepoxide was given; 15 min later subjects were injected with either abecarnil or flumazenil, and 15 min later they were tested for lever selection. As these tests were repeated over the next several days, flumazenil substitution for PTZ was lost and abecarnil never substituted for chlordiazepoxide. *n*, 15 and 16 for abecarnil and flumazenil, respectively

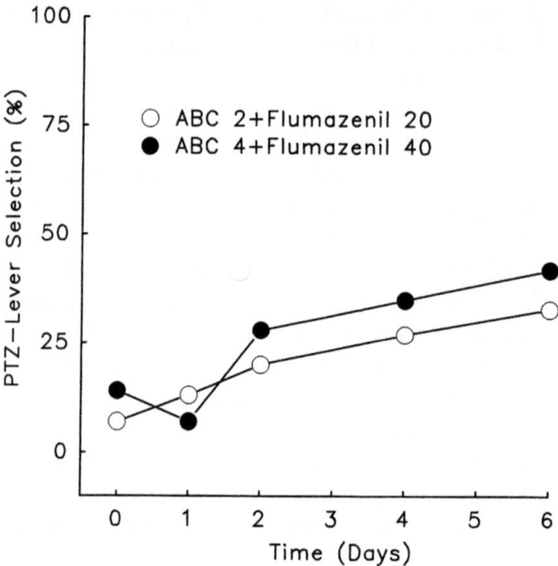

Fig. 4. Failure of flumazenil to substitute for PTZ during chronic administration of abecarnil (*ABC*). *Ordinate*, see Fig. 1. *Abscissa*, number of days of chronic abecarnil administration. Abecarnil (2 or 4 mg/kg, i.p.) was given every 8 h. Tests occurred 8 h after a preceding injection of abecarnil, thus subjects were injected with their regularly scheduled dose of abecarnil. 15 min later they were injected with flumazenil and 15 min after flumazenil, they were tested. *n*, 15 and 14 for the 2 and 4 mg/kg groups, respectively

days. When tested with flumazenil during this 6-day period, vehicle lever selection occurred in both groups (Fig. 4).

3 Flumazenil Cue in Dependent Rats

In this paradigm, 15 rats were trained to discriminate flumazenil (2.5 mg/kg) from carboxymethylcellulose vehicle using the same technique described for PTZ training. However, additionally, the rats were maintained chronically on chlordiazepoxide, which was given in two oral feedings each day. Subjects received 25 mg/kg of the daily dose of chlordiazepoxide in a nutritionally complete liquid diet (Lal et al. 1988), which was given 6 h prior to training. The remaining 75 mg/kg of the daily dose of chlordiazepoxide was given in the liquid diet immediately following each training session. In this discrimination, subjects were maintained on the liquid diet containing chlordiazepoxide for at least 2 weeks before any training started, and at the conclusion of experiments that tested for time course of spontaneous withdrawal, they were reinstated on the diet for at least 2 weeks before training was resumed.

In subjects maintained on chronic chlordiazepoxide and trained to detect flumazenil, abecarnil did not substitute for flumazenil (Table 1). Upon termination of chronic chlordiazepoxide and testing with vehicle, the subjects initially selected the flumazenil lever (Fig. 5). Over the next 10–14 days, vehicle testing produced lever selection that shifted progressively from the flumazenil to the vehicle lever; in addition, at the end of these tests, PTZ still produced flumazenil-lever selection. The substitution of vehicle for flumazenil that occurred 24 h after termination of chronic chlordiazepoxide

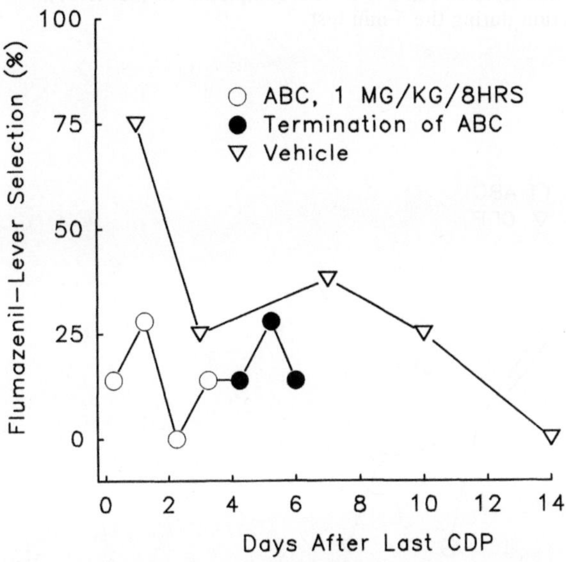

Fig. 5. Time course of substitution of vehicle for flumazenil following termination of chronic chlordiazepoxide (*CDP*) and effect of abecarnil (*ABC*) administration on this time course. *Ordinate*, percent of subjects selecting the flumazenil lever (0 indicates all subjects selected the vehicle lever). *Abscissa*, time since the last administration of chlordiazepoxide in the liquid diet. Subjects were maintained on a chronic liquid diet containing 100 mg/kg chlordiazepoxide. Six hours after a feeding containing 25 mg/kg chlordiazepoxide, they were trained to discriminate flumazenil (2.5 mg/kg) from vehicle. Subjects were given a final feeding of chlordiazepoxide and then tested with vehicle at the indicate times. On day 18, a substitution test with 20 mg/kg PTZ was conducted. Initially, vehicle substituted for flumazenil, but by day 14, vehicle administration again produced full vehicle-lever selection. When tested with the training dose of flumazenil on day 14 (data not shown), subjects selected the vehicle lever. PTZ still substituted fully for flumazenil at a time (18 days) when flumazenil no longer produced flumazenil selection (data not shown), supporting the hypothesis that this discrimination trains subjects to detect a PTZ-like stimulus that is only produced by flumazenil when subjects are maintained chronically on chlordiazepoxide. In contrast to the results obtained, when subjects were terminated from chlordiazepoxide and left untreated, when 1 mg/kg abecarnil was given every 8 h starting at the time chlordiazepoxide was discontinued, the vehicle lever was selected in all tests over the next 3 days. When abecarnil was then discontinued, the vehicle lever continued to be selected. Thus, with abecarnil treatment, no evidence of benzodiazepine withdrawal was obtained. For all tests $n = 8$

Table 1. Failure of abecarnil to substitute for flumazenil in rats maintained chronically on chlordiazepoxide (100 mg/kg per day) and trained to detect flumazenil (2.5 mg/kg)[a]

Abecarnil (mg/kg)	Flumazenil-level selection (%)	Number of subjects[b]
0.10	14	7
0.33	0	9
1.00	11	9
3.30	11	9

[a] Abecarnil was given 15 min prior to testing. Subjects were allowed to respond for up to 5 min or until one of the levers was selected (an FR 10 was completed on that lever).
[b] All subjects made a lever selection during the 5-min test.

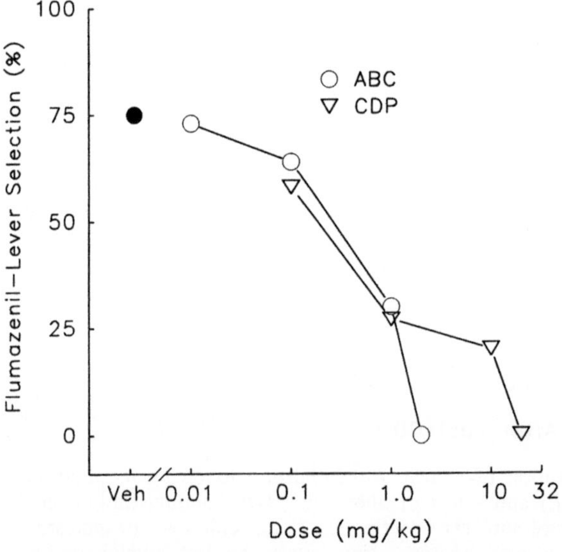

Fig. 6. Blockade of spontaneous withdrawal from chlordiazepoxide (∇) by chlordiazepoxide and abecarnil ($\bigcirc$). A flumazenil-like stimulus occurs with vehicle tests performed 24 h after terminating chronic chlordiazepoxide. This substitution of vehicle for the flumazenil-training stimulus was blocked in a dose-dependent manner by both chlordiazepoxide and abecarnil

was blocked by chlordiazepoxide or abecarnil in a dose-dependent manner (Fig. 6). In a final experiment, chronic chlordiazepoxide was halted, and beginning 8 h after the last feeding of chlordiazepoxide, treatment was initiated with abecarnil, 1 mg/kg per 8 h. In contrast to the results in Fig. 5 for vehicle tests after chlordiazepoxide was halted, when these subjects were tested with vehicle 8 h postabecarnil on days 1, 2, and 3 following termination of chlordiazepoxide, predominantely vehicle-lever selection occurred (Fig. 5); in addition, when abecarnil was then terminated, tests with vehicle continued to produce predominately vehicle-lever selection.

4 Discussion

Abecarnil was fully effective in blocking the PTZ stimulus, as was chlordiazepoxide, a known anxiolytic drug. Because of the utility of the PTZ discrimination in identifying anxiolytic drugs (Lal and Emmett-Oglesby 1983), the present data are consistent with the suggestion of Stephens et al. (1990) that abecarnil is an anxiolytic. Stephens et al. (1990) also observed that abecarnil blocks the PTZ stimulus, and the present observation that flumazenil, a benzodiazepine-receptor antagonist, prevents this blocking action of abecarnil is consistent with the hypothesis that the mechanism of action of abecarnil involves binding at the benzodiazepine-receptor site.

The tests of dependence in these experiments are based upon the observation that when given acutely, the benzodiazepine antagonist, flumazenil, does not substitute for PTZ, but following chronic administration of a fully efficacious benzodiazepine agonist, flumazenil does substitute for PTZ (for a review, see Emmett-Oglesby et al. 1990). In the present experiment, when a fully efficacious benzodiazepine agonist (chlordiazepoxide) was administered for a week, flumazenil substituted for PTZ. These data are consistent with previous reports from this laboratory in which chronic administration of another benzodiazepine, diazepam, resulted in flumazenil substitution for PTZ within 48 h of starting diazepam administration (Emmett-Oglesby et al. 1987). In contrast to those results with benzodiazepines, when flumazenil was tested at various times after starting chronic abecarnil, either 2 or 4 mg/kg per 8 h, flumazenil failed to produce significant PTZ-lever selection over 6 days of chronic abecarnil administration. These data suggest that abecarnil has significantly less potential for producing dependence than classical benzodiazepines. Because these results were obtained from an animal model of subjective phenomena they extend the conclusions reached in observational models of dependence/withdrawal in which abecarnil was also found to have much less potential for producing dependence than full benzodiazepine-receptor agonists (Sannerud et al. 1992; see also chapters by Sannerud et al. by Löscher, by Serra et al. and by Stephens et al.).

In receptor assays, binding of ligands at the benzodiazepine site is modified by the addition of gamma-aminobutyric acid (GABA) to the assay (Braestrup et al. 1982). When GABA is added to the assay, the binding affinity of inverse agonists is decreased, the binding affinity of full agonists is enhanced, and the binding of pure antagonists is not affected (for a review, see Stephens et al. 1987). Abecarnil binding is only slightly increased by the addition of GABA to the binding medium (Stephens et al. 1990), which has been the basis for the suggestion that abecarnil is a partial agonist (Stephens et al. 1990). Is a partial agonist activity of abecarnil the reason why this drug seems to produce less dependence than a drug such as chlordiazepoxide? Although this question cannot be answered with assurance, the evidence from these experiments do not suggest a partial agonist effect of abecarnil. First, abecarnil was fully efficacious in blocking the PTZ cue. Perhaps more importantly, we can argue by analogy to the opioid literature that abecarnil does not produce effects consistent with those expected of a partial agonist. In opioid pharmacology, when subjects dependent upon full agonists are treated with partial agonists, withdrawal is precipitated (Jaffe 1990). Thus, if abecarnil were a partial agonist, one might expect that it would precipitate withdrawal from benzodiazepine dependence. In two tests, that was not the case in these experiments. First, in the PTZ discrimination, in subjects dosed chronically with the full agonist chlordiazepoxide, flumazenil substituted for PTZ; in contrast, abecarnil failed to substitute for PTZ in subjects maintained on chlordiazepoxide. Second, in animals maintained on chronic chlordiazepoxide and trained to discriminate flumazenil, abecarnil failed to substitute for flumazenil. Based upon these data, we suggest that abecarnil is likely to have the profile of a fully efficacious anxiolytic (see also chapter by Stephens et al.). Thus, abecarnil should not unmask dependence when given to patients who have been taking high doses of benzodiazepines on a chronic basis.

In subjects treated chronically with chlordiazepoxide and trained to discriminate flumazenil, the results of this study suggest that flumazenil produces a cue that is PTZ like in character, that flumazenil only produces this cue in dependent subjects, and that if chlordiazepoxide is discontinued, a flumazenil-like stimulus spontaneously arises, with a readily measured time course of 10–14 days over which it disappears. These data support the hypothesis that this discrimination is based upon a cue related to withdrawal from benzodiazepine dependence. In this model, abecarnil blocks spontaneous withdrawal in a dose-related fashion. In addition, if abecarnil is given every 8 h following termination of chronic chlordiazepoxide, it suppresses spontaneous withdrawal over the 3 days that it was administered; upon termination of abecarnil after this 3-day period, spontaneous withdrawal appeared to be largely over since no occurrence of a stimulus like the flumazenil training stimulus was detected by these subjects. These data suggest that abecarnil may be useful for weaning patients from benzodiazepine dependence by minimizing subjective aspects of benzodiazepine withdrawal while producing little dependence of its own.

It is with some trepidation that we offer the suggestion that abecarnil may be useful for weaning subjects from dependence upon benzodiazepines. There are few examples of drugs that are useful for treating drug withdrawal without the danger of simply substituting one drug of dependence for another. Particularly if abecarnil is anxiolytic by acting through the same receptor mechanisms as benzodiazepines, it would be all the more remarkable that this drug should suppress benzodiazepine withdrawal without producing a dependence of its own. It may turn out to be the case that the dosing regimen or some other feature of our experimental paradigm accounts for the failure to see withdrawal. Nonetheless, our initial data support the utility of abecarnil as a novel treatment for benzodiazepine withdrawal.

Acknowledgments. Supported by NIDA grant R01-3521.

References

Braestrup C, Schmiechen R, Neef G, Nielsen M, Petersen EN (1982) Interaction of convulsive ligands with benzodiazepine receptors. Science 216:1241–1243

Emmett-Oglesby MW, Rowan GA (1991) Drug discrimination used to study drug withdrawal. In: Glennon RA, Jarbe TUC, Frankenheim J (eds) NIDA Research Monograph 116: Drug discrimination: application to drug abuse research. US Department of Health and Human Services, ADAMHA, Rockville, Maryland, pp 337–357

Emmett-Oglesby MW, Mathis DA, Lal H (1987) Diazepam tolerance and withdrawal assessed in an animal model of subjective drug effects. Drug Dev Res 11:145–156

Emmett-Oglesby MW, Mathis DA, Moon RTY, Lal H (1990) Animal models of drug withdrawal symptoms. Psychopharmacology 101:292–309

Jaffe J (1990) Drug addiction and drug abuse. In: Gilman AG, Rail TW, Nies AS, Taylor P (eds) Goodman and Gilman's: the pharmacological basis of therapeutics. Pergamon, New York, pp 535–539

Lal H, Emmett-Oglesby MW (1983) Animal models of anxiety. Neuropharmacology 22:1423–1441

Lal H, Harris CM, Benjamin D, Springfield AC, Bhadra S, Emmett-Oglesby MW (1988) Characterization of a pentylenetetrazol-like interoceptive stimulus produced by ethanol withdrawal. J Pharmacol Exp Ther 247:508–518

Preston KL, Bigelow GE (1991) Subjective and discriminative effects of drugs. Behav Pharmacol 2:293–313

Sannerud CA, Ator NA, Griffiths RR (1992) Behavioral pharmacology of abecarnil in baboons: self-administration, drug discrimination and physical dependence. Behav Pharmacol (in press)

Stephens DN, Schneider HH, Kehr W, Jensen LH, Petersen E, Honore T (1987) Modulation of anxiety by betacarbolines and other benzodiazepine-receptor ligands: relationship of pharmacological to biochemical measures of efficacy. Brain Res Bull 19:309–318

Stephens DN, Schneider HH, Kehr W, Andrews JS, Rettig K-J, Turski L, Schmiechen R, Turner JD, Jensen LH, Petersen EN, Honore T, Bondo-Hansen J (1990) Abecarnil, a metabolically stable, anxioselective beta-carboline acting at benzodiazepine receptors. J Pharmacol Exp Ther 253:334–343

Abecarnil: A New ß-Carboline Anxiolytic Preliminary Clinical Pharmacology

T. DUKA, W. KRAUSE, R. DOROW, A. ROHLOFF, H. OTT, and B. VOET

1 Introduction

Benzodiazepines have been the treatment of choice for anxiety because of their high efficacy and good safety profile (for review, see Rickels 1983; Dommisse and Hayes 1987). However, their depressant effects on the central nervous system (CNS), expressed as sedation, ataxia and often amnesia, as well as their dependence potential after long-term use, often complicate the course of the treatment.

On the basis of these considerations, pharmacologists have directed their research to developing substances which possess some benzodiazepine effects, i.e., anxiolytic, anticonvulsant, but lack others, i.e., sedative, amnesic. Among such compounds are the ß-carboline-3-carboxylic-acid ester derivatives (ß-carbolines) which cover with their pharmacological activities the whole spectrum of benzodiazepine effects as demonstrated in animal (Petersen 1983; Stephens and Kehr 1985; Petersen and Jensen 1984; Jensen et al. 1984) and human studies (Dorow et al. 1983; Duka et al. 1987, 1988; Dorow et al. 1987a,b; Moller et al. 1990). Unfortunately the poor bioavailability of these compounds precluded their clinical development and directed further efforts to synthesising stable substances with similar pharmacological properties (Krause et al. 1989).

Abecarnil (isopropyl-6-benzyloxy-4-methoxymethyl-ß-carboline-3-carboxylate) is one of a series of such compounds with good metabolic stability as demonstrated in monkeys (Krause and Mengel 1990) and with high affinity for benzodiazepine receptors. The ideal profile of abecarnil, as manifested in studies of its pharmacological activity in preclinical pharmacology (Stephens et al. 1990; Turski et al. 1990), its effects during spontaneous and precipitated withdrawal in different animal species after longterm treatment (Löscher et al. 1990; Sannerud et al. 1992), and its pharmacokinetic properties suggested that abecarnil would be an appropriate candidate for development as an anxiolytic. In the following, the initial pharmacokinetic studies, part of the Phase I programme will be reviewed, including the tolerability, safety and initial pharmacological profile of abecarnil, as well as

Research Laboratories, Schering AG, Berlin and Bergkamen, Germany the antagonism of its effects by the benzodiazepine antagonist flumazenil; furthermore, the initial investigation in patients will be presented. Data from these trials will be discussed in the light of abecarnil's selective properties at the benzodiazepine receptors.

2 Preliminary Pharmacological Characterisation of Abecarnil After Single and Multiple Administration

In a classical Phase I approach, the safety and tolerability of abecarnil in increasing doses was assessed in two double-blind, placebo-controlled trials (a single- and a multiple-dose trial). In the single-dose trial, the increasing doses of abecarnil administered to different groups of ten volunteers (seven verum; three placebo) were 1 mg, 5 mg, 10 mg, 20 mg and 40 mg per os. The second trial, a multiple-dose trial, had as its increasing doses 15 mg (5 mg tid), 30 mg (10 mg tid), 60 mg (20 mg tid) and 90 mg (30 mg tid). These doses were administered over 7 days (days 1–7). In order to study the pharmacokinetics of abecarnil after single administration and in steady state, abecarnil was given as a single dose in the morning of the 1st and 7th day of treatment, and plasma was sampled at 0.5, 1, 1.5, 2, 3, 4, 6, 9, 12 and 15 h after drug administration. One day before treatment was initiated (baseline; day 0) and 2 days after discontinuation of treatment (follow up; days 8–9), placebo was administered in a single blind fashion. In both trials at certain time points before and after treatment, evaluations were performed to estimate safety, tolerability and drug effects. For single doses up to 40 mg and for multiple doses up to 30 mg tid, abecarnil was found to be safe and well-tolerated. Adverse events were observed with doses of 20 mg and 40 mg in the single-dose trial, and with the 20 mg tid and 30 mg tid in the multiple-dose trial. The most frequently occurring adverse events when compared to placebo in both trials were dizziness and equilibrium loss (unsteady gait); drowsiness (sleepiness) or marked sedation were not observed or reported by the volunteers. For further details see Duka et al. 1993.

To estimate drug effects related to sedation and psychomotor performance, in the single-dose trial visual analogue scales (VAS) the digit symbol substitution task (DSST) were used 30 min before drug administration, and at 1.5, 3.5, 5.5 and 24 h post dose. In the multiple-dose trial, the same tests were employed on days 0–9, 2.5 h after the morning dose. The VAS, a bipolar scale with the opposing poles "sleepy" (0) and "alert" (100), was used to investigate sedative or stimulant drug effects, since volunteers were asked to consider the midpoint as representing their normal mood state and to mark the scale spontaneously at the point which they felt best corresponded to their current mood. During performance on the DSST (Wechsler 1955), volunteers were presented with a series of digits and asked to copy symbols coded to the digits 1 to 9 as quickly and as correctly as

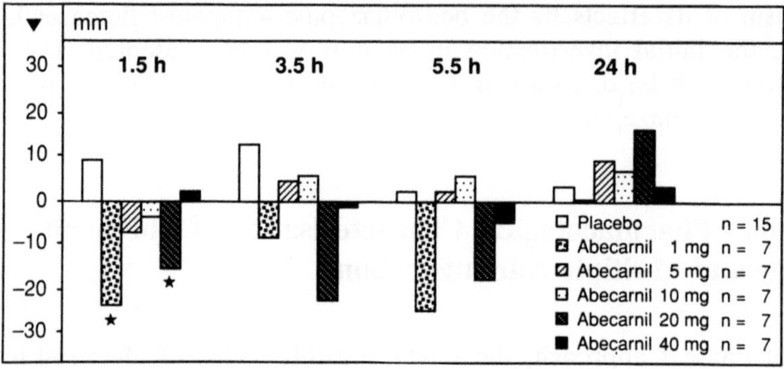

Fig. 1. Time course of self-rating (visual analogue scale; 0, sleepy; 100, alert) changes after different single doses or abecarnil; values above 0 indicate subjective feeling of alertness and below 0 of sleepiness; values at each time point were subtracted from baseline values (shortly before treatment); $*p < 0.05$, compared with placebo

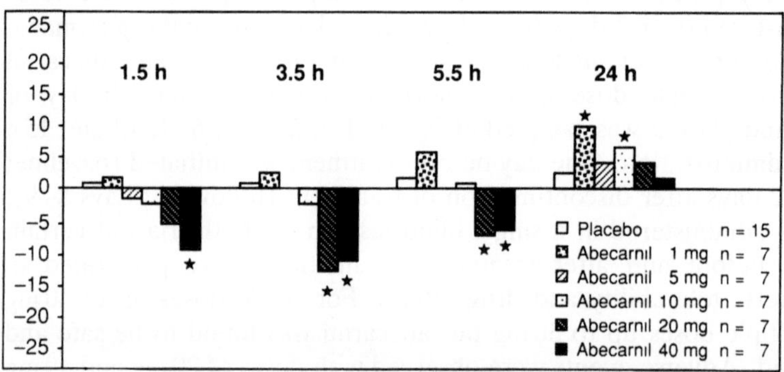

Fig. 2. Time course of changes in performance on digit symbol substitution task after different single doses of abecarnil; values above 0 indicate improvement and below from baseline values (shortly before treatment). $*p < 0.05$, compared with placebo

possible within 90 s. This test was employed to detect psychomotor effects of the drug related especially to visuomotor coordination, although changes in working memory functions and attentional processes could also affect task performance.

A divergence was found between changes induced by abecarnil on VAS (Fig. 1) and DSST (Fig. 2) in the single-dose trial. In the doses at which abecarnil impaired performance in the DSST, it did not influence volunteers' alertness as evidenced by the VAS. As can be seen in Fig. 1, self ratings did not indicate sleepiness except at the doses of 1 mg and 20 mg 1.5 h after treatment. However, in the DSST, 40 mg abecarnil impaired performance 1.5, 3.5 and 5.5 h after treatment and 20 mg impaired it 3.5 and 5.5 h after treatment, when compared with placebo (Fig. 2). This effect was attributable to a decrease in the number of correct answers, while no effects on answers made in errors (accuracy) were seen (data not shown).

Peak drug effects documented by measurements of performance in DSST (Fig. 1) were seen 1.5–3.5 h after drug administration, whereas performance was returning to normal 5.5 h post treatment, a time course which coincides with the plasma levels time course of abecarnil (see also Krause et al. 1990). It is interesting that at the low doses (1–10 mg single or 5 mg tid multiple) at which moderate abecarnil plasma concentration had been measured (see also Krause et al. 1990), the effects of abecarnil on DSST were mild and noted only sporadically.

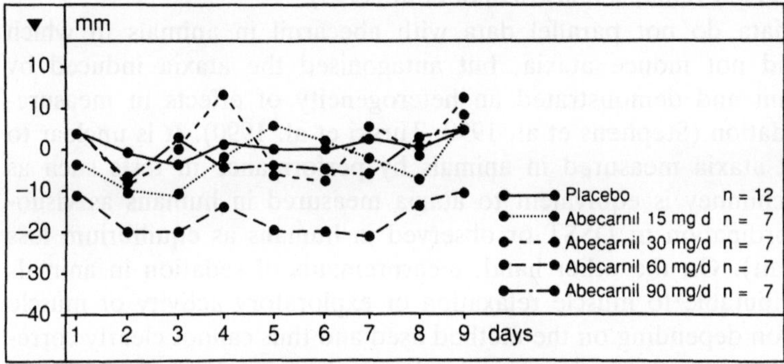

Fig. 3. Time course of self-rating (visual analogue scale) changes after different multiple doses of abecarnil; values above 0 indicate subjective feeling of alertness and below 0 of sleepiness; values of each day were subtracted from baseline values (day 0); (ANOVA, not significant)

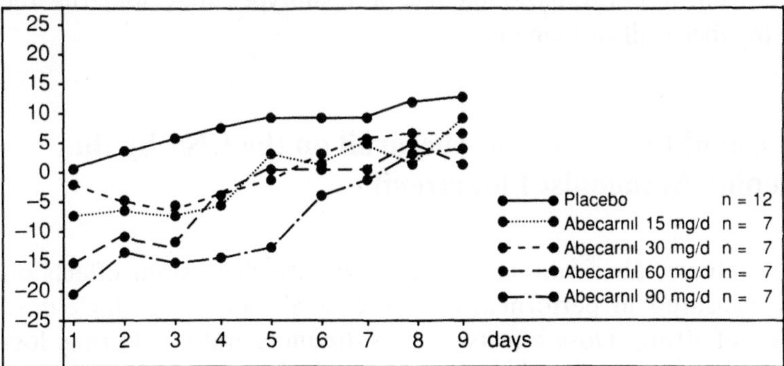

Fig. 4. Time course of changes in performance in the digit symbol substitution task after different multiple doses of abecarnil; values above 0 indicate improvement and below 0 impairment of performance; values of each day were subtracted from baseline values (day 0). Significant differences were found (ANOVA, $p < 0.05$) between placebo and all the other treatments on days 2–6 and between placebo and 60 mg/day, 90 mg/day on day 7 of treatment

A similar divergence of abecarnil effects on VAS and DSST was found during repeated treatment (7 days; Figs. 3, 4). Again, abecarnil did not alter significantly the state of volunteers' alertness except at the dose 20 mg tid. However, performance in DSST was impaired significantly in a dose-dependent fashion from the 2nd day of treatment with all doses of abecarnil tested, but persisted only with doses of 20 mg and 30 mg tid. Changes in performance were attributed to a decrease in number of correct responses whereas accuracy (number of errors) was not affected (data not shown).

These data have suggested a divergence of abecarnil effects, i.e., impairment of psychomotor performance (DSST) and incidence of dizziness and/or equilibrium loss (unsteady gait), but lack of marked sedation (reports of adverse events; see also Duka et al. 1993).

These data do not parallel data with abecarnil in animals in which abecarnil did not induce ataxia, but antagonised the ataxia induced by lormetazepam and demonstrated an heterogeneity of effects in measurements of sedation (Stephens et al. 1990; Turski et al. 1990). It is unclear to what extent ataxia measured in animals by performance in tests such as rotarod or chimney is equivalent to ataxia measured in humans as visuo-motor incoordination in DSST or observed in humans as equilibrium loss (unsteady gait). On the other hand, measurements of sedation in animals may be attributable to muscle relaxation or exploratory activity or muscle incoordination depending on the method used and thus cannot clearly correspond to measurement of subjective sedation in humans. It can be assumed that they are controlled by different neurophysiological mechanisms. Thus it may be difficult to interpret the present data in light of the animal findings. Nevertheless, at doses at which performance in DSST was impaired and unsteadiness was observed, no marked sedation was rated by the subjects or observed by the trial staff. It is unclear and very speculative whether selectivity of abecarnil at benzodiazepine receptor subtypes may underlie the effects seen by abecarnil in humans.

3 Antagonism of the Effects of Abecarnil on the CNS by the Benzodiazepine Antagonist Flumazenil

As mentioned above, abecarnil was found to induce depressant effects on the CNS as measured in performance on the DSST following single-dose administration of 20 mg. Dose effects such as dizziness and equilibrium loss (unsteady gait) have also been documented in this dose. Since the purpose of this trial was to ascertain the efficacy of flumazenil as an antidote for abecarnil overdose, a single dose of 20 mg abecarnil was administered, although at that stage of development, abecarnil was known to show efficacy in a much lower dose (1–3 mg tid; Ballenger et al. 1991). The aim in using three different doses of flumazenil was to ascertain the minimum effective dose of this compound as an antagonist for abecarnil. Furthermore this trial should provide information about safety in the use of abecarnil in clinical investigations, during which cases of overdose cannot be excluded.

All 16 healthy male volunteers who participated in the trial received 20 mg abecarnil per os and 2 h later intravenously either placebo or 0.3, 0.9, or 2.7 mg flumazenil in a double-blind four times cross-over design (Duka et al. 1990). Objective measurements of sedation, cognitive functions, steadiness and psychomotor performance were taken. Only data obtained from the actograph, which was used for an objective measurement of steadiness, and from the DSST will be presented here.

At the high dose, abecarnil tested in combination with either 0.3, 0.9, or 2.7 mg flumazenil was found to be safe and well-tolerated. The abecarnil-induced impairment in balance seen in the values obtained after treatment was not observed when abecarnil was combined with 2.7 mg flumazenil (Fig. 5), indicating an antagonistic effect only at the high dose of flumazenil ($p < 0.05$, when differences from baseline were compared between placebo and this dose). Failure of flumazenil at the low doses (0.3 mg, 0.9 mg) to antagonise this effect of a high dose of abecarnil (20 mg) indicates that

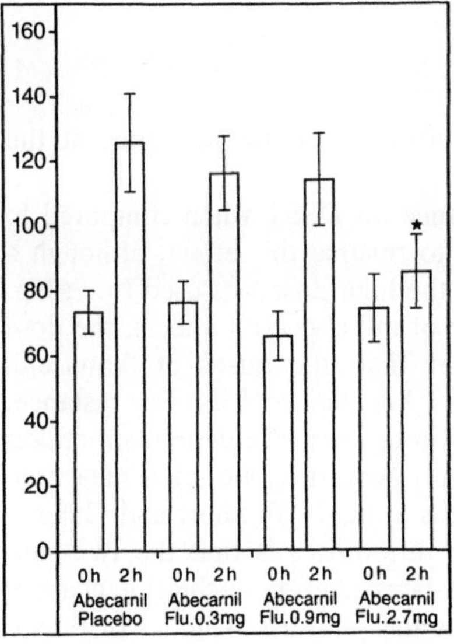

Fig. 5. Maximum deviations ($N = kg\,m/s^2$) from baseline position (0 line) in 20 s on the actograph before and after different treatment combinations. ANOVA, $p = 0.007$; *LSD procedure, $p < 0.1$ compared with placebo. In this balance test, 16 volunteers were required to stand on a platform (actograph), and their body movements were registered as maximum deviations from the 0 line (baseline position) within 20 s expressed as force in Newton: $N = kg\,m/s^2$; volunteers had their eyes closed, outstretched arms and palms facing upwards, feet close together and the legs straight (steadiness known as Romberg's sign). The right foot was on the measuring platform, the left on a fixed platform next to it

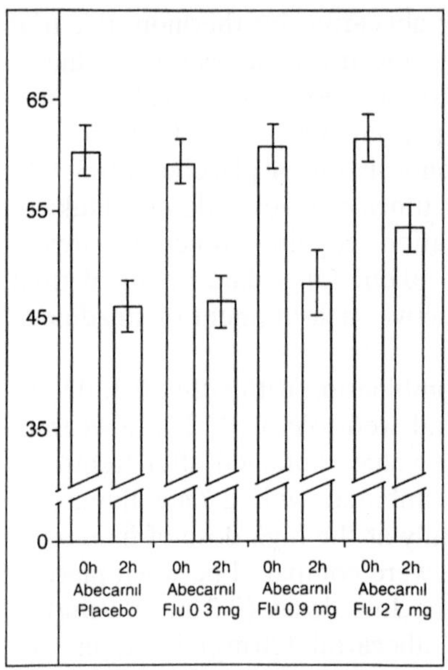

Fig. 6. Number of correct answers in DSST before and after different treatment combinations (ANOVA, $p = 0.112$, n.s.)

this dose probably leads to a high concentration of the substance at the receptor site.

Abecarnil also impaired the performance on DSST when compared to baseline values. Flumazenil was not able to reverse this effect, although a slight antagonism could be detected when the high dose was used (n.s.; Fig. 6). Although flumazenil antagonised some of the abecarnil effects, the dose of flumazenil needed seems to be higher than the doses of flumazenil required to antagonise the effects of known benzodiazepines. For instance, 1 mg flumazenil i.v. was able to completely antagonise the depressant effects of midazolam (a full benzodiazepine receptor agonist hypnotic) as measured by psychomotor tests including DSST (Ochs et al. 1990; Short and Galletly 1989). One possible explanation of these differences is that the two substances interact differently with the GABA-benzodiazepine-chloride channel receptor complex. A more likely reason is the pharmacokinetics of flumazenil: the half-life of flumazenil in plasma is approximately 60 min (Klotz et al. 1985) and the measurements took place between 10 and 50 min after drug administration. Since actograph and DSST measurements took place 20 and 40 min after flumazenil injection, respectively, differences in plasma concentration of flumazenil may be the basis for the differences in potencies. However, a different test sensitivity cannot be excluded. In future trials, these questions can be addressed directly and may be clarified.

4 Pharmacokinetics of Abecarnil

In the multiple dose trial in which safety and tolerability were tested (see Sect. 2) single- and multiple-dose pharmacokinetics of abecarnil were also investigated. Blood samples were collected following the morning dose on the 1st and 7th day, respectively, at 0.5, 1, 1.5, 2, 3, 4, 6, 9, 12 and 15 h. For the treatment schedule, see Sect. 2. In addition blood samples were drawn prior to the morning dose during the treatment days, in order to evaluate trough drug level under steady state conditions. Pharmacokinetics of abecarnil after single dose and in steady state can be compared in Table 1. These data show that absorption of all doses of abecarnil was relatively rapid ($t_{1/2} = 0.5$) and peak plasma levels were reached after 1–3 h and did not change under steady state conditions. The terminal half-life of abecarnil also remained unchanged in the range from 5 to 7 h.

Both after single administration or under steady state conditions there was a dose-proportional increase in C_{max}. When trough levels were examined, a slight accumulation of drug was observed; steady state was achieved on the 3rd day, except with the 90 mg/day dose during which steady state was reached on day 4 (Fig. 7). It may be that absorption is delayed when the dose applied is high, as can also be seen from the increase of t_{max} in the highest dose. In another trial, the biotransformation of abecarnil (Krause et al. 1991) was tested in eight elderly volunteers who first received an i.v. injection of 1.88 mg (86 μCi) and 2 weeks later an oral dose of 10.3 mg (101 μCi) of ^{14}C-labelled abecarnil.

Table 1. Pharmacokinetic parameters after single (a) and multiple (b) application of abecarnil in different doses

Treatment days	Pharmacokinetic parameters	15 mg/day (5 mg tid)	30 mg/day (10 mg tid)	60 mg/day (20 mg tid)	90 mg/day (30 mg tid)
Day 1 (a)		$n = 7$	$n = 7$	$n = 7$	$n = 7$
	C_{max} (ng/ml)	9.2 ± 5.0	8.5 ± 4.3	16.0 ± 10.0	21.0 ± 7.0
	t_{max} (h)	1.9 ± 0.7	2.1 ± 1.8	2.6 ± 1.9	2.6 ± 0.9
	AUC_{0-24} (h ng/ml)	72.8 ± 40.8	60.0 ± 48.6	148.0 ± 80.6	201.1 ± 76.5
	$t_{1/2}$ (a) (h)	–	1.9 ± 0.3	–	–
	$t_{1/2}$ (b) (h)	4.9 ± 1.4	6.5 ± 2.2	7.0 ± 1.6	6.7 ± 2.3
Day 7 (b)		$n = 5$	$n = 7$	$n = 6$	$n = 7$
	C_{max} (ng/ml)	16.0 ± 8.3	21.0 ± 15.0	42.0 ± 28.0	49.0 ± 19.0
	t_{max} (h)	1.1 ± 0.4	1.5 ± 0.7	1.4 ± 0.4	$2.5 \pm 0.9^*$
	AUC_{0-24} (h ng/ml)	107.0 ± 53.0	199.0 ± 173.0	317.0 ± 267.0	425.0 ± 211.0
	$t_{1/2}$ (a) (h)	–	–	–	–
	$t_{1/2}$ (b) (h)	4.5 ± 1.9	6.5 ± 1.00	5.5 ± 1.3	4.7 ± 0.9

$^*p < 0.05$ (versus all the other doses)

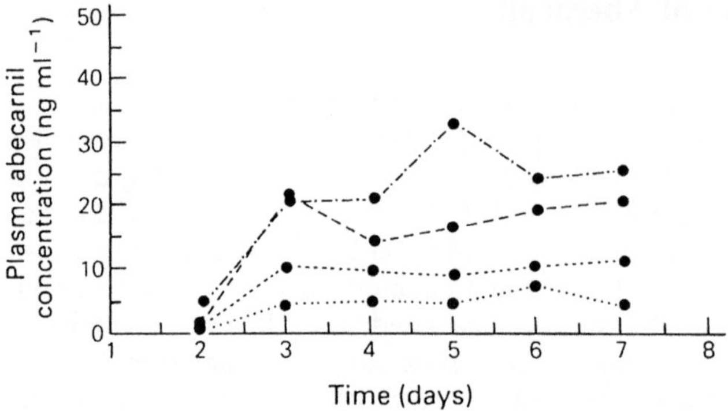

Fig. 7. Trough plasma concentrations of abecarnil prior to each morning dose during the 5 days of t.i.d. dosing

Table 2. Pharmacokinetic parameters and elimination of ^{14}C-labelled compounds in eight healthy male volunteers after i.v. injection and oral administration of ^{14}C adecarnil

	Intravenous injection		Oral administration	
	Mean $\pm$ SD	Range	Mean $\pm$ SD	Range
Plasma (^{14}C)				
C_{max} (ng equiv/ml)	84 $\pm$ 21	59–120	95 $\pm$ 16	62–112
t_{max} (h)	0.05	0.05	1.2 $\pm$ 0.4	1–2
AUC (h ng equiv/ml)	101 $\pm$ 34	55–149	263 $\pm$ 478	392–1675
Cl_{tot} (ml/min per kg)	4.3 $\pm$ 1.9	2.4 $\pm$ 8.1	–	–
$t_{1/2}$ (1) (h)	<0.05	<0.05	0.4 $\pm$ 0.2	0.1–0.8
$t_{1/2}$ (2) (h)	4.8 $\pm$ 1.8	2.2–7.2	22 $\pm$ 11	8–38
Urine (^{14}C)				
Excretion (% dose)	24.6 $\pm$ 3.9	17.0–35.3	22.2 $\pm$ 4.3	16.9–31.3
$t_{1/2}$ (h)	10.4 $\pm$ 4.3	4.7–18.2	15.6 $\pm$ 5.0	9.6–23.8
Faeces (^{14}C)				
Excretion (% dose)	58.9 $\pm$ 20.0	24.8–94.5	57.9 $\pm$ 11.8	31.5–67.7
$t_{1/2}$ (h)	15.4 $\pm$ 7.0	7.8–24.8	14.6 $\pm$ 4.9	10.6–23.6
Recovery (% dose)	83.5 $\pm$ 21.5	44.9–113.8	80.0 $\pm$ 13.2	48.4–89.1
Faeces (drug)				
Excretion (% dose)	2.1 $\pm$ 0.7	1.0–2.7	9.6 $\pm$ 3.3	4.4–14.6

Data are mean values $\pm$ SD of $n = 8$ and range. Oral dose of ^{14}C-abecarnil was 10.3 mg and i.v. dose was 1.88 mg.

In Table 2, the pharmacokinetic parameters and elimination of ^{14}C-labelled compounds can be seen, and in Table 3 the same parameters for unchanged abecarnil are given. The metabolite patterns as estimated in this trial can be seen in Fig. 8.

When the urinary elimination of labelled compounds after oral and i.v. administration were compared (Table 2), the extent of absorption was cal-

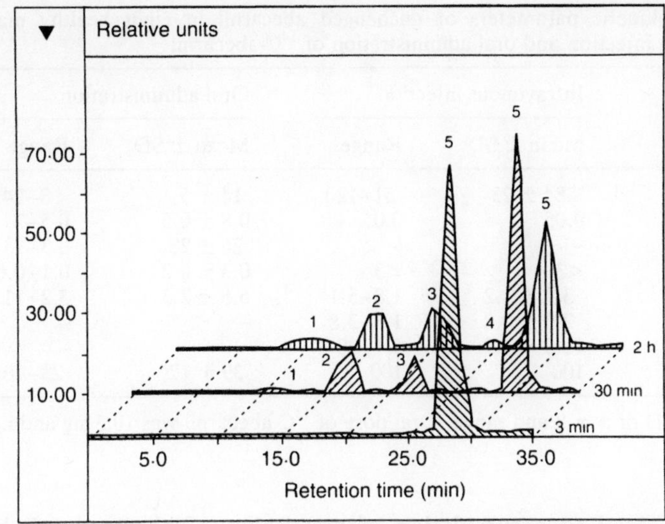

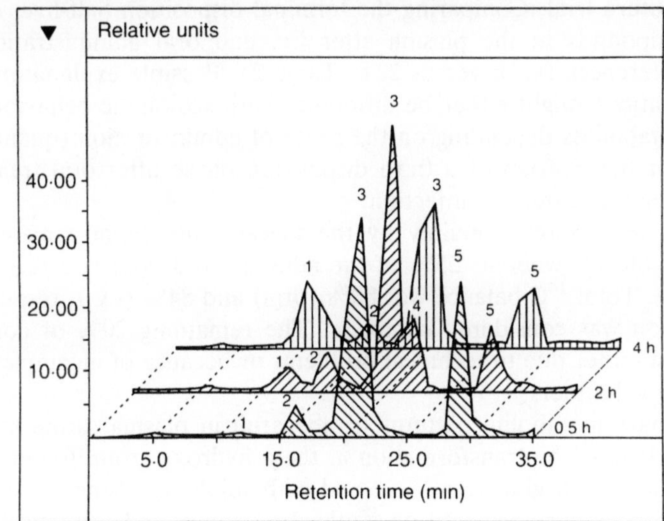

Fig. 8a,b. Metabolite patterns obtained by radio-hplc of plasma of eight healthy male volunteers after intravenous injection (**a**) or oral administration (**b**) of ^{14}C

culated as 90 ± 20%. Due to the relatively high first-pass effect, metabolite patterns in the plasma were quantitatively different after i.v. and oral treatment (Fig. 8), so that absorption cannot be calculated from an area under the curve (AUC) comparison of ^{14}C activity in the plasma.

^{14}C-Labelled compounds exhibited a much longer disposition half-life in the plasma than the unchanged drug (22 h versus 6.6 h; Tables 2, 3), especially after oral treatment. Multiple oral dosing using a tid regimen

Table 3. Pharmacokinetic parameters of unchanged abecarnil in eight healthy male volunteers after i.v. injection and oral administration of ^{14}C-abecarnil

	Intravenous injection		Oral administration	
	Mean ± SD	Range	Mean ± SD	Range
C_{max} (ng/ml)	84 ± 23	51–120	14 ± 5	8–24
t_{max} (h)	0.05	0.05	0.8 ± 0.5	0.5–2
$t_{1/2}$ abs. (min)	–	–	26 ± 28	3–73
$t_{1/2}$ (1) (min)	<3	<3	0.3 ± 0.2	0.1–0.6
$t_{1/2}$ (2) (h)	3.7 ± 1.2	1.8–5.1	6.6 ± 2.3	3.2–11.1
V_{ss} (1/kg)	2.6 ± 0.8	1.6–3.8	–	–
Cl_{tot} (ml/min per kg)	11.3 ± 4.3	5.7–20.0	–	–
Bioavailability (%)	100	100	39 ± 17	23–70

Data are mean ± SD of n = 8 and range. Oral dose of ^{14}C-abecarnil was 10.3 mg and i.v. dose 1.88 mg.

should therefore lead to accumulation of metabolites. This issue will be addressed in a future trial. Comparing the terminal disposition half-lives of ^{14}C-labelled compounds in the plasma after i.v. and oral administration reveals great differences (4.8 h versus 22 h; Table 2). Possible explanations for these observations might either be different pharmacokinetic behaviour of individual metabolites depending on the route of administration (quantitative aspects) or the overlap of a third disposition phase after oral treatment which is not seen after i.v. injection.

^{14}C-Activity was excreted mainly by the faecal route (approximately 60% of dose; Table 2), whereas 25% of the administered dose was recovered in the urine. Total ^{14}C balance was 80% (oral) and 84% (i.v.), respectively. Elimination was considered complete. The remaining 20% of dose was probably lost either due to technical problems or because of incomplete collection by the volunteers.

The preliminary metabolite patterns of abecarnil in plasma, urine and faeces indicated Phase I biotransformation at the 6-hydroxy group followed by conjugation both with glucuronic acid and with sulphate. Using cochromatography with previously isolated or synthesized compounds, practically all metabolites of abecarnil could tentatively be identified. At present, tests on pharmacological and toxicological activity of these metabolites are in progress.

5 The First Clinical Trial with Abecarnil in Generalized Anxiety Disorders

Based on the data from Phase I trials (Duka et al. 1993) in healthy volunteers, indicating a safe profile of abecarnil, the first clinical trial was initiated in outpatients with generalised anxiety disorders (Ballenger et al. 1991). Primary objectives of the trial were to investigate safety and tolerability of multiple doses of abecarnil, the secondary objectives were to obtain preliminary evidence of efficacy. In a sequential dose-finding design, three dose ranges, 15–30 mg/day, 7.5–15 mg/day, and 3–9 mg/day, were compared with placebo. All doses were given tid. A fixed dosage regimen (forced titration) was used for the 1st week and increases were made over the next 2 weeks to attain the doses outlined in Table 4. In the 3–9 mg/day group, the dose was doubled after the 1st week and further increased to 9 mg in the 3rd week.

A total of 129 patients were allocated randomly to treatment groups and received at least one dose of trial medication; for group size and patient disposition into different treatments, see Table 4. Safety measurements (ECG, vital signs, laboratory parameters) indicated that abecarnil was safe in all doses used. A number of adverse CNS events were reported in the high-dose group. Because of this, the original dosage schedule had been amended to allow for two lower dosage ranges, i.e. medium dose and low dose instead of the originally planned dosage increase of 30–60 mg/day and 60–90 mg/day. The most frequent adverse events drowsiness and equilibrium loss (unsteady gait) appeared to be dose-related. Adverse events were frequently found in the 15–30 mg dose, whereas occurrence of adverse events in the 3–9 mg group was not very different from the placebo group. The frequency of adverse events for all treatments is presented in Table 5.

In the main efficacy variables, Clinical Global Impression scale (CGI) and the Hamilton Anxiety scale (HAM-A) abecarnil was found to be better than placebo. In CGI, which assesses the severity of the patient's illness, abecarnil (3–9 mg/day group) was better than placebo at week 3, whereas in the CGI for the patient's overall improvement, abecarnil in the same group

Table 4. Number of patients with generalized anxiety disorders and mean dose (mg) of abecarnil per week of treatment

Treatment group	Week 1	Week 2	Week 3
15–30 mg per day			
n	34	28	24
dose	13.7	20.2	21.4
7.5–15 mg			
n	35	34	33
dose	6.6	12	12.2
3–9 mg per day			
n	32	32	32
dose	2.9	5.5	7.7
Placebo			
n	28	27	27
dose	–	–	–

Table 5. Percentage of patients with generalized anxiety disorders with the most frequently occurring central nervous system side effects during treatment with abecarnil

Side effects	15–30 mg ($n = 34$)	7.5–15 mg ($n = 35$)	3–9 mg ($n = 32$)	Placebo ($n = 28$)
Drowsiness	71	51	31	14
Equilibrium loss (unsteady gait)	26	11	6	0
Confusion	24	3	3	0
Dizziness	18	11	3	11
Fatigue	15	17	12	0
Coordination difficulty	12	14	3	0

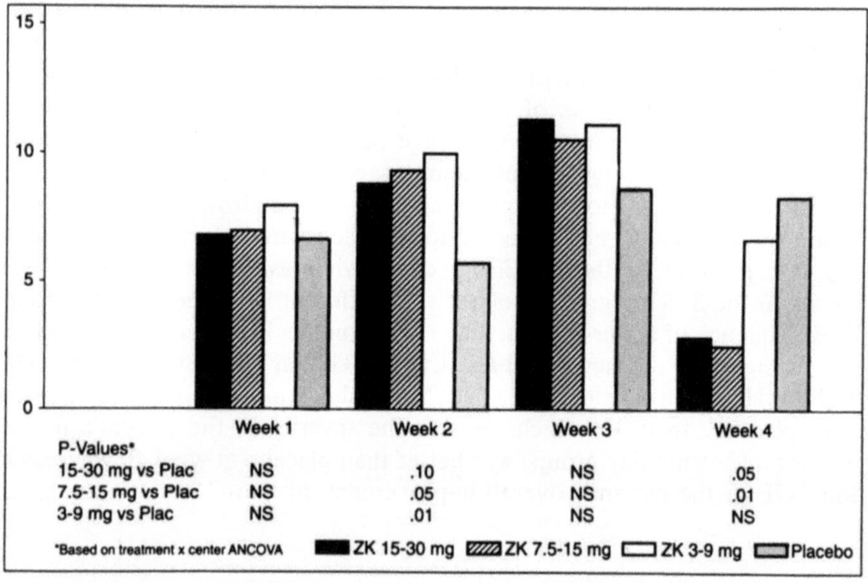

Fig. 9. Hamilton anxiety scale total: mean changes from baseline (higher is better; *ZK*, abecarnil). (With permission from Ballenger et al. 1991)

was better than placebo in weeks 2 and 3 (Ballenger et al. 1991). HAM-A consists of 14 items, each of which is rated on a five-point scale from 0 (not present) to 4 (very severe); data on the evaluation of efficacy using HAM-A can be seen in Fig. 9. Abecarnil in the low dose range was significantly superior to placebo at the $p < 0.05$ level (two-tailed) analysis of covariance for the HAM-A total (week 2).

In summary, the first dose-finding study of abecarnil demonstrated a dosage range that is both safe and efficacious. The 3–9 mg/day dose not only showed superior efficacy to placebo, but also had an acceptable adverse reaction profile. For the two higher doses, adverse events in some patients given 15–30 mg/day would preclude the use of starting doses as high as 15 mg/day; the 7.5–15 mg/day dose, while more efficacious, still caused adverse events at 15 mg/day (Table 5). The results of this trial have been reported in full by Ballenger et al. 1991. The positive outcome of this study is especially notable given the constraints placed upon the design, the fact that it was a multicentre study, the small size of the treatment groups and the high placebo response. This first dose-finding study of abecarnil resulted in the selection of a dose range for further trials designed to test clinically the very promising results obtained here; it also appears probable that the optimal dose range for an expanded programme of phase II trials with abecarnil has been established. For instance, the 3–9 mg/day dose not only showed superior efficacy to placebo but also had an acceptable adverse reaction profile. Thus this trial with its exploratory character has offered useful information for planning future abecarnil studies and choosing appropriate doses and has provided reasonable preliminary evidence of the safety and efficacy of abecarnil in generalised anxiety disorders.

6 General Discussion

In the present review, an effort has been made to outline the pharmacological profile of abecarnil, as characterised up until now in human volunteer trials. Early data on the efficacy of abecarnil in patients with generalised anxiety have also been presented. Whereas doses between 3 and 9 mg/day of abecarnil were efficacious compared with placebo in counteracting symptoms of generalised anxiety, doses of abecarnil as high as 90 mg/day have been tolerated in healthy volunteers with only moderate depressant effects on the CNS. These were expressed mostly as equilibrium loss (unsteady gait) in volunteers and drowsiness in patients. Thus there was a discrepancy between the incidence of adverse events in the two different populations, patients and normal volunteers. One possible reason is the difference in the way adverse events were documented in the two trials, e.g., original documentation in different languages (in the volunteer trial, the original language was German).

Nevertheless, in both populations, CNS side effects were seen only at high doses. This wide separation of abecarnil doses with anxiolytic properties (in the patient trial) and of doses with CNS depressant effects (in the patient and in the healthy volunteer trial) is consistent with partial agonist properties of abecarnil. However some other data presented in this review may indicate selective agonistic activity, e.g., the separation between the effect of abecarnil on alertness as measured by the VAS and on psychomotor performance as measured by carrying out the DSST. Nevertheless, the available data are not yet sufficient to allow us to draw any conclusions about abecarnil's pharmacological profile in humans.

References

Ballenger JC, McDonald S, Noyes R, Rickels K, Sussman N, Woods S, Patin J, Singer J (1991) The first double-blind, placebo controlled trial of a partial benzodiazepine agonist abecarnil (ZK 112-119) in generalized anxiety disorder. Psychopharmacol Bull 27:171–179

Dommisse CS, Hayes PE (1987) Current concepts in clinical therapeutics: anxiety disorders, part 2. Clin Pharm 6:196–215

Dorow R, Horowski R, Paschelke G, Amin M, Braestrup C (1983) Severe anxiety induced by FG 7142, a β-carboline ligand for benzodiazepine receptors. Lancet II:98

Dorow R, Duka T, Höller L, Sauerbrey N (1987a) Clinical perspectives of β-carbolines from first studies in humans. Brain Res Bull 19:319–326

Dorow R, Duka T, Sauerbrey N, Höller L (1987b) β-carbolines: New insights into the clinical pharmacology of benzodiazepine receptor ligands. In: Dahl S, Gram LF, Paul SM, Potter WZ (eds) Clinical pharmacology in psychiatry: selectivity in psychotropic drug action – promises or problems. Psychopharmacology [Suppl. 3]:37–51

Duka T, Stephens DN, Krause W, Dorow R (1987) Studies on the benzodiazepine receptor antagonist β-carboline ZK 93 426: preliminary observations on the psychotropic activity. Psychopharmacology 93:421–427

Duka T, Goerke D, Dorow R, Höller L, Fichte K (1988) Human studies on the benzodiazepine receptor antagonist β-carboline ZK 93 426: antagonism of lormetazepam's psychotropic effects. Psychopharmacology 95:463–471

Duka T, Schütt B, Mager T, Dorow R, Mc Donald S, Ott H (1990) Abecarnil, a β-carboline anxiolytic: phase I studies to establish safety, tolerability and drug effects. CINP (Abstracts) 1:147

Duka T, Schütt B, Krause W, Dorow R, McDonald S, Fichte K (1993) Human studies on Abecarnil a new β-carboline anxiolytic: safety, tolerability and preliminary pharmacological profile. Br J Clin Pharmacol 35:386–394

Jensen LH, Petersen EN, Braestrup C, Honore T, Kehr W, Stephens DN, Schneider HH, Seidelmann D, Schmiechen R (1984) Evaluation of the β-carboline ZK 93 426 as a benzodiazepine receptor antagonist. Psychopharmacology 83:349–356

Klotz U, Duka T, Dorow R, Doenicke A (1985) Flunitrazepam and lormetazepam do not affect the pharmacokinetics of the benzodiazepine antagonist Ro 15-1788. Br J Clin Pharmacol 26:95–98

Krause W, Mengel H (1990) Pharmacokinetics of the anxiolytic β-carboline derivative, abecarnil, in the mouse, the rat, the rabbit, the dog, the cynomologous monkey and the baboon. Studies on species differences. Drug Res 40:522–529

Krause W, Mengel H, Nordholm L (1989) Determination of β-carboline derivatives in biological samples by high-performance liquid chromatography with fluorescence detection. J Pharmaceut Sci 78:622–626

Krause W, Schütt B, Duka T (1990) Pharmacokinetics and acute tolerability of the β-carboline derivative ZK 112 119 in man. Arzeimittel Forsch 40:529–532

Krause W, Duka T, Matthes H (1991) Pharmacokinetics and biotransformation of the anxiolytic abecarnil in healthy volunteers. Xenobiotica 21:763–774

Löscher W, Hönack D, Scherkl R, Hashem A, Frey HH (1990) Pharmakokinetics, anticonvulsant efficacy and adverse effects of the β-carboline abecarnil a novel ligand of benzodiazepine receptors, after acute and chronic administration in dogs. J Pharmacol Exp Ther 255:541–548

Moller A, Jensen LH, Skrumsager B, Blatt-Lyon B, Pedersen B, Dam M (1990) Inhibition of photosensitive seizures in man by the β-carboline, ZK 95962, a selective benzodiazepine receptor agonist. Epilepsy Res 5:155–159

Ochs MW, Tucker MR, Owsley TG, Anderson JA (1990) The effectiveness of flumazenil in reversing the sedation and amnesia produced by intravenous midazolam. J Oral Maxillofac Surg 48:240–245

Petersen EN (1983) DMCM: A potent convulsive benzodiazepine receptor ligand. Eur J Pharmacol 94:117–124

Petersen EN, Jensen LH (1984) Proconflict effect of benzodiazepine receptor inverse agonists and other inhibitors of GABA function. Eur J Pharmacol 103:91–97

Rickels K (1983) Benzodiazepines in the treatment of anxiety: North American experiences. In: Costa E (ed) The benzodiazepines: from molecular biology to clinical practice. Raven, New York, pp 295–310

Sannerud C, Ator NA, Griffiths RR (1992) Behavioural pharmacology of abecarnil in baboons: self injection, drug discrimination and physical dependence. Behav Pharmacol 3:507–516

Short TG, Galletly D (1989) Residual psychomotor effects following reversal of midazolam sedation with flumazenil. Anaesth Intens Care 17:290–297

Stephens DN, Kehr W (1985) β-carbolines can enhance or antagonize the effects of punishment in mice. Psychopharmacology 85:143–174

Stephens DN, Schneider HH, Kehr W, Andrews JS, Rettig KJ, Turski L, Schmiechen R, Turner JD, Jensen LH, Petersen EN, Honore T, Bondo Hansen J (1990) Abecarnil, a metabolically stable anxioselective β-carboline acting at benzodiazepine receptors. J Pharmacol Exp Ther 253:334–343

Turski L, Stephens DN, Jensen LH, Petersen EN, Meldrum BS, Patel S, Bondo Hansen J, Löscher W, Schneider HH, Schmiechen R (1990) Anticonvulsant action of the β-carboline Abecarnil – studies in rodents and baboon, Papio papio. J Pharmacol Exp Ther 253:344–352

Wechsler D (1955) Adult Intelligence Scales: a manual. Psychological Corporation, New York

Subject Index